# Healthy Sleep

## Recent Titles in Q&A Health Guides

# HEALTHY SLEEP

## Your Questions Answered

John T. Peachey and Diane C. Zelman

**Q&A Health Guides**

BLOOMSBURY ACADEMIC

NEW YORK • LONDON • OXFORD • NEW DELHI • SYDNEY

BLOOMSBURY ACADEMIC
Bloomsbury Publishing Inc
1385 Broadway, New York, NY 10018, USA
50 Bedford Square, London, WC1B 3DP, UK
29 Earlsfort Terrace, Dublin 2, Ireland

BLOOMSBURY, BLOOMSBURY ACADEMIC and the Diana logo are trademarks of
Bloomsbury Publishing Plc

First published in the United States of America 2023

**Library of Congress Cataloging in Publication Control Number: 2023007391**

ISBN: HB: 978-1-4408-7885-5
ePDF: 978-1-4408-7886-2
eBook: 979-8-216-17171-3

Series: Q&A Health Guides

Typeset by Amnet ContentSource
Printed and bound in the United States of America

To find out more about our authors and books visit www.bloomsbury.com and sign up for
our newsletters.

This book is dedicated to Mary Carskadon, and other pioneering researchers in child, adolescent, and young adult sleep.

# Contents

# Series Foreword

All of us have questions about our health. Is this normal? Should I be doing something differently? Whom should I talk to about my concerns? And our modern world is full of answers. Thanks to the Internet, there's a wealth of information at our fingertips, from forums where people can share their personal experiences to Wikipedia articles to the full text of medical studies. But finding the right information can be an intimidating and difficult task—some sources are written at too high a level, others have been oversimplified, while still others are heavily biased or simply inaccurate.

*Q&A Health Guides* address the needs of readers who want accurate, concise answers to their health questions, authored by reputable and objective experts, and written in clear and easy-to-understand language. This series focuses on the topics that matter most to young adult readers, including various aspects of physical and emotional well-being as well as other components of a healthy lifestyle. These guides will also serve as a valuable tool for parents, school counselors, and others who may need to answer teens' health questions.

All books in the series follow the same format to make finding information quick and easy. Each volume begins with an essay on health literacy and why it is so important when it comes to gathering and evaluating health information. Next, the top five myths and misconceptions that surround the topic are dispelled. The heart of each guide is a collection of questions and answers, organized thematically. A selection of five case studies provides real-world examples to illuminate key concepts. Rounding out each volume are a directory of resources, glossary, and index. It is our hope that the books in this series will not only provide valuable information but will also help guide readers toward a lifetime of healthy decision making.

# Acknowledgments

We give special thanks to Maxine Taylor, for her support and encouragement throughout the writing process, and gratitude and love for our families, who tolerated the writing process.

Diane Zelman thanks her husband Michael, their children Mira, Saul, and Zane, and dear friends Barbara Hollinger and Jim Rebhan, for their support of Diane's writing and fascination with sleep.

# Introduction

Sleep is the ideal medicine for overall wellness. Getting enough good quality sleep results in healthy brain and body functioning as well as a longer life and better quality of life. On the other hand, a lack of sleep is devastating to human health, sometimes fatally so. When medical and mental health problems arise, people often fail to consider the role of sleep in causing or continuing the problem. Modern cultures that prioritize work and play over sleep ("I'll sleep when I'm dead") tend to ignore or undervalue sleep's critical importance, mistakenly viewing sleepiness as a weakness to be overcome rather than an undeniable daily experience. Undoubtedly, a lack of education on sleep has contributed to this misunderstanding, which this book aims to correct.

When adults sleep less than seven hours nightly, or teens less than nine hours, every system in the body suffers. When sleep deprived, we become physically weaker and slower, performing worse in sports or physical labor. Our thinking is slowed too, with more difficulties in remembering, learning, and paying attention that can interfere with school, work, and emergency response. A lack of sleep causes the immune system to become less effective—we get sick more easily, respond less effectively to vaccines, and die younger than our well-slept peers. Unusual nighttime experiences like nightmares and sleepwalking (also called parasomnias) also occur more often when we are sleep deprived.

Sleep loss can lead to irritability and relationship difficulties, as well as loss of attractiveness (e.g., sagging skin, weight gain). Sexual fitness often suffers too, as sleep loss lowers sexual drive, decreases sex hormones, and reduces sperm count and testicle size in men. All of these difficulties can contribute to stress and mood complications, although poor or insufficient sleep can itself lead to more mental health problems like depression or anxiety.

Those with medical conditions, mental health concerns, or poor quality of life typically report more difficulties sleeping. On the other hand, unluckily, disturbances of sleep cause more physical and emotional problems. Given this, one could argue that any effective health treatment plan should include efforts to improve sleep quality, as ignoring sleep can undermine recovery from medical concerns. Sleep researcher Matthew Walker echoed this position when he stated, "Sleep is the greatest legal performance enhancing drug that most people are probably neglecting." And it's true—good health and quality sleep go hand in hand. Unlike most medications, the miracle drug of sleep is free, natural, and easily obtainable and it has minimal side effects.

The purpose of this book is to answer common questions that many people ask about sleep (e.g., Why am I sleepy all the time?) as well as to address common misperceptions and myths about sleep and dreaming (e.g., I can't get to sleep until midnight—isn't that normal for teenagers?). Using commonly asked questions (e.g., Why do we dream?), the book begins with an overview of the basics of sleep and dreaming. Next, the book explores the connection between sleep, learning and memory, mental and physical health, relationships, and athletic performance. Questions about sleep disorders and common sleep difficulties are then introduced with concise and easy-to-understand explanations.

Unfortunately, there is an ongoing lack of sleep services and professionals in many areas, including places where our readers may reside. Turning to the nearly bottomless pit of bad advice online is unlikely to help. So, the final portion of this book aims to fill this gap by providing practical tips and strategies for independently improving your sleep. The book ends with case examples that demonstrate important sleep concerns and how they are treated, a glossary of terms, and a directory of resources to further guide readers.

Sleep Well.

# Guide to Health Literacy

On her 13th birthday, Samantha was diagnosed with type 2 diabetes. She consulted her mom and her aunt, both of whom also have type 2 diabetes, and decided to go with their strategy of managing diabetes by taking insulin. As a result of participating in an after-school program at her middle school that focused on health literacy, she learned that she can help manage the level of glucose in her bloodstream by counting her carbohydrate intake, following a diabetic diet, and exercising regularly. But, what exactly should she do? How does she keep track of her carbohydrate intake? What is a diabetic diet? How long should she exercise and what type of exercise should she do? Samantha is a visual learner, so she turned to her favorite source of media, YouTube, to answer these questions. She found videos from individuals around the world sharing their experiences and tips, doctors (or at least people who have "Dr." in their YouTube channel names), government agencies such as the National Institutes of Health, and even video clips from cat lovers who have cats with diabetes. With guidance from the librarian and the health and science teachers at her school, she assessed the credibility of the information in these videos and even compared their suggestions to some of the print resources that she was able to find at her school library. Now, she knows exactly how to count her carbohydrate level, how to prepare and follow a diabetic diet, and how much (and what) exercise is needed daily. She intends to share her findings with her mom and her aunt, and now she wants to create a chart that summarizes what she has learned that she can share with her doctor.

Samantha's experience is not unique. She represents a shift in our society; an individual no longer views himself or herself as a passive recipient of medical care but as an active mediator of his or her own health. However, in this era when any individual can post his or her opinions and experiences with a particular health condition online with just a few clicks or publish a memoir, it is vital that people know how to assess the credibility of health information. Gone are the days when "publishing" health information required intense vetting. The health information landscape is highly saturated, and people have innumerable sources where they can find information about practically any health topic. The sources (whether print, online, or a person) that an individual consults for health information are crucial because the accuracy and trustworthiness of the information can potentially affect his or her overall health. The ability to find, select, assess, and use health information constitutes a type of literacy—health literacy—that everyone must possess.

## THE DEFINITION AND PHASES OF HEALTH LITERACY

One of the most popular definitions for health literacy comes from Ratzan and Parker (2000), who describe health literacy as "the degree to which individuals have the capacity to obtain, process, and understand basic health information and services needed to make appropriate health decisions." Recent research has extrapolated health literacy into health literacy bits, further shedding light on the multiple phases and literacy practices that are embedded within the multifaceted concept of health literacy. Although this research has focused primarily on online health information seeking, these health literacy bits are needed to successfully navigate both print and online sources. There are six phases of health information seeking: (1) Information Need Identification and Question Formulation, (2) Information Search, (3) Information Comprehension, (4) Information Assessment, (5) Information Management, and (6) Information Use.

The first phase is the *information need identification and question formulation phase*. In this phase, one needs to be able to develop and refine a range of questions to frame one's search and understand relevant health terms. In the second phase, *information search*, one has to possess appropriate searching skills, such as using proper keywords and correct spelling in search terms, especially when using search engines and databases. It is also crucial to understand how search engines work (i.e., how search results are derived, what the order of the search results means, how to use the snippets that are provided in the search results list to select websites, and how to determine which listings are ads on a search engine results page). One also has to limit reliance on surface characteristics, such as the design of a website or a book (a website or book that appears to have a lot of information or looks aesthetically pleasant does not necessarily mean it has good information) and language used (a website or book that utilizes jargon, the keywords that one used to conduct the search, or the word "information" does not necessarily indicate it will have good information). The next phase is *information comprehension*, whereby one needs to have the ability to read, comprehend, and recall the information (including textual, numerical, and visual content) one has located from the books and/or online resources.

To assess the credibility of health information (*information assessment* phase), one needs to be able to evaluate information for accuracy, evaluate how current the information is (e.g., when a website was last updated or when a book was published), and evaluate the creators of the source—for example, examine site sponsors or type of sites (.com, .gov, .edu, or .org) or the author of a book (practicing doctor, a celebrity doctor, a patient of a specific disease, etc.) to determine the believability of the person/organization providing the information. Such credibility perceptions tend to become generalized, so they must be frequently reexamined (e.g., the belief that a specific news agency always has credible health information needs continuous vetting). One also needs to evaluate the credibility of the medium (e.g., television, Internet, radio, social media, and book) and evaluate—not just accept without questioning—others' claims regarding the validity of a site, book, or other specific source of information. At this stage, one has to "make sense of information gathered from diverse sources by identifying misconceptions, main and supporting ideas, conflicting information, point of view, and biases" (American Association of School Librarians [AASL], 2009, p. 13) and conclude which sources/information are valid and accurate by using conscious strategies rather than simply using intuitive judgments or "rules of thumb." This phase is the most challenging segment of health information seeking and serves as a determinant of success (or lack thereof) in the information-seeking process. The following section on Sources of Health Information further explains this phase.

The fifth phase is *information management*, whereby one has to organize information that has been gathered in some manner to ensure easy retrieval and use in the future. The last phase is *information use*, in which one will synthesize information found across various resources, draw conclusions, and locate the answer to his or her original question and/or the content that fulfills the information need. This phase also often involves implementation, such as using the information to solve a health problem; make health-related decisions; identify and engage in behaviors that will help a person to avoid health risks; share the health information found with family members and friends who may benefit from it; and advocate more broadly for personal, family, or community health.

## THE IMPORTANCE OF HEALTH LITERACY

The conception of health has moved from a passive view (someone is either well or ill) to one that is more active and process based (someone is working toward preventing or managing disease). Hence, the dominant focus has shifted from doctors and treatments to patients and prevention, resulting in the need to strengthen our ability and confidence (as patients and consumers of health care) to look for, assess, understand, manage, share, adapt, and use health-related information. An individual's health literacy level has been found to predict his or her health status better than age, race, educational attainment, employment status, and income level (National Network of Libraries of Medicine, 2013). Greater health literacy also enables individuals to better communicate with health care providers such as doctors, nutritionists, and therapists, as they can pose more relevant, informed, and useful questions to health care providers. Another added advantage of greater health literacy is better information-seeking skills, not only for health but also in other domains, such as completing assignments for school.

## SOURCES OF HEALTH INFORMATION: THE GOOD, THE BAD, AND THE IN-BETWEEN

For generations, doctors, nurses, nutritionists, health coaches, and other health professionals have been the trusted sources of health information. Additionally, researchers have found that young adults, when they have health-related questions, typically turn to a family member who has had firsthand experience with a health condition because of their family member's close proximity and because of their past experience with, and trust in, this individual. Expertise should be a core consideration when consulting a person, website, or book for health information. The credentials and background of the person or author and conflicting interests of the author (and his or her organization) must be checked and validated to ensure the likely credibility of the health information they are conveying. While books often have implied credibility because of the peer-review process involved, self-publishing has challenged this credibility, so qualifications of book authors should also be verified. When it comes to health information, currency of the source must also be examined. When examining health information/studies presented, pay attention to the exhaustiveness of research methods utilized to offer recommendations or conclusions. Small and nondiverse sample size is often—but not always—an indication of reduced credibility. Studies that confuse correlation with causation is another potential issue to watch for. Information seekers must also pay attention to the sponsors of the research studies. For example, if a study is sponsored by manufacturers of drug Y and the study recommends that drug Y is the best treatment to manage or cure a disease, this may indicate a lack of objectivity on the part of the researchers.

The Internet is rapidly becoming one of the main sources of health information. Online forums, news agencies, personal blogs, social media sites, pharmacy sites, and celebrity "doctors" are all offering medical and health information targeted to various types of people in regard to all types of diseases and symptoms. There are professional journalists, citizen journalists, hoaxers, and people paid to write fake health news on various sites that may appear to have a legitimate domain name and may even have authors who claim to have professional credentials, such as an MD. All these sites *may* offer useful information or information that appears to be useful and relevant; however, much of the information may be debatable and may fall into gray areas that require readers to discern credibility, reliability, and biases.

While broad recognition and acceptance of certain media, institutions, and people often serve as the most popular determining factors to assess credibility of health information among young people, keep in mind that there are legitimate Internet sites, databases, and books that publish health information and serve as sources of health information for doctors, other health sites, and members of the public. For example, MedlinePlus (https://medlineplus.gov) has trusted sources on over 975 diseases and conditions and presents the information in easy-to-understand language.

The chart here presents factors to consider when assessing credibility of health information. However, keep in mind that these factors function only as a guide and require continuous updating to keep abreast with the changes in the landscape of health information, information sources, and technologies.

The chart can serve as a guide; however, approaching a librarian about how one can go about assessing the credibility of both print and online health information is far more effective than using generic checklist-type tools. While librarians are not health experts, they can apply and teach patrons strategies to determine the credibility of health information.

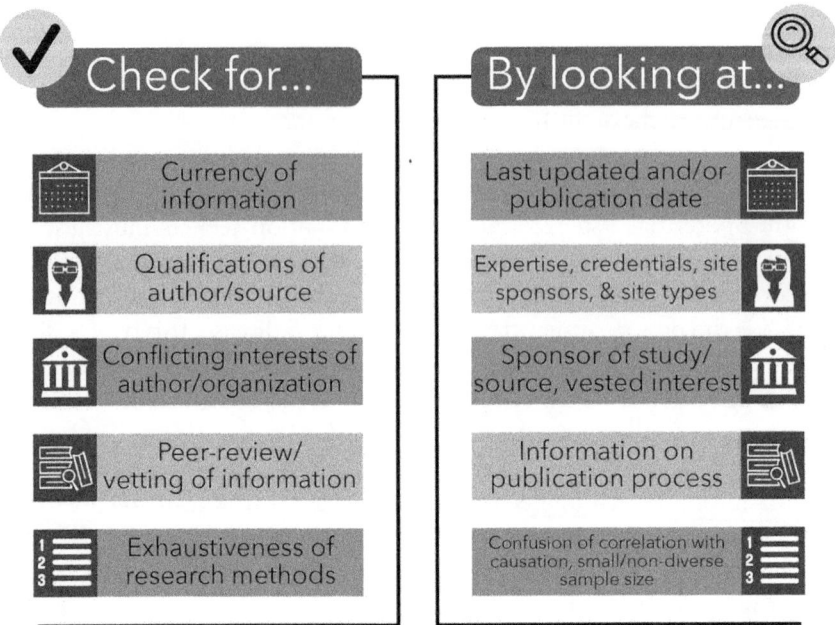

All images from flaticon.com

With the prevalence of fake sites and fake resources that appear to be legitimate, it is important to use the following health information assessment tips to verify health information that one has obtained (St. Jean et al., 2015, p. 151):

- **Don't assume you are right**: Even when you feel very sure about an answer, keep in mind that the answer may not be correct, and it is important to conduct (further) searches to validate the information.
- **Don't assume you are wrong**: You may actually have correct information, even if the information you encounter does not match—that is, you may be right and the resources that you have found may contain false information.
- **Take an open approach**: Maintain a critical stance by not including your preexisting beliefs as keywords (or letting them influence your choice of keywords) in a search, as this may influence what it is possible to find out.
- **Verify, verify, and verify**: Information found, especially on the Internet, needs to be validated, no matter how the information appears on

the site (i.e., regardless of the appearance of the site or the quantity of information that is included).

Health literacy comes with experience navigating health information. Professional sources of health information, such as doctors, health care providers, and health databases, are still the best, but one also has the power to search for health information and then verify it by consulting with these trusted sources and by using the health information assessment tips and guide shared previously.

Mega Subramaniam, PhD
Associate Professor, College of Information Studies,
University of Maryland

## REFERENCES AND FURTHER READING

American Association of School Librarians (AASL). (2009). *Standards for the 21st-century learner in action.* Chicago, IL: American Association of School Librarians.

Hilligoss, B., & Rieh, S.-Y. (2008). Developing a unifying framework of credibility assessment: Construct, heuristics, and interaction in context. *Information Processing & Management, 44*(4), 1467–1484.

Kuhlthau, C. C. (1988). Developing a model of the library search process: Cognitive and affective aspects. *Reference Quarterly, 28*(2), 232–242.

National Network of Libraries of Medicine (NNLM). (2013). Health literacy. Bethesda, MD: National Network of Libraries of Medicine. Retrieved from nnlm.gov/outreach/consumer/hlthlit.html

Ratzan, S. C., & Parker, R. M. (2000). Introduction. In C. R. Selden, M. Zorn, S. C. Ratzan, & R. M. Parker (Eds.), *National Library of Medicine current bibliographies in medicine: Health literacy.* NLM Pub. No. CBM 2000–1. Bethesda, MD: National Institutes of Health, U.S. Department of Health and Human Services.

St. Jean, B., Taylor, N. G., Kodama, C., & Subramaniam, M. (February 2017). Assessing the health information source perceptions of tweens using card-sorting exercises. *Journal of Information Science.*Retrieved from http://journals.sagepub.com/doi/abs/10.1177/0165551516687728

St. Jean, B., Subramaniam, M., Taylor, N. G., Follman, R., Kodama, C., & Casciotti, D. (2015). The influence of positive hypothesis testing on youths' online health-related information seeking. *New Library World, 116*(3/4), 136–154.

Subramaniam, M., St. Jean, B., Taylor, N. G., Kodama, C., Follman, R., & Casciotti, D. (2015). Bit by bit: Using design-based research to improve the health literacy of adolescents. *JMIR Research Protocols*, 4(2), paper e62. Retrieved from http://www.ncbi.nlm.nih.gov/pmc /articles/PMC4464334/

Valenza, J. (2016, November 26). Truth, truthiness, and triangulation: A news literacy toolkit for a "post-truth" world [Web log]. Retrieved from http://blogs.slj.com/neverendingsearch/2016/11/26/truth-truthiness-triangulation-and-the-librarian-way-a-news-literacy-toolkit-for-a -post-truth-world/

# Common Misconceptions about Healthy Sleep

## 1. WE CAN CATCH UP ON LOST SLEEP BY NAPPING OR SLEEPING IN ON THE WEEKENDS

When we fail to meet our sleep need—which for teenagers usually falls between 8 and 10 hours—we build up a "sleep debt." While it may be tempting to nap or sleep in on the weekends to pay off this debt, this often makes the problem worse by preventing us from finding a consistent sleep schedule. Alternatively, "banking" or saving up sleep in advance of expected periods of sleep loss is equally unlikely to work. These strategies cannot make up for lost sleep and often interfere in other major ways. Short naps of 20–30 minutes do provide a temporary improvement in concentration, but naps do nothing to address problems in learning, memory, emotional regulation, and physical functioning following sleep loss. Napping also increases the risk of difficulties in falling asleep at night. This is because, as happens with snacking before a meal, the body becomes less "hungry" for sleep at bedtime because the nap "snack" reduces the natural pressure (or appetite) to sleep. Unfortunately, we don't pay back our debt equally where one hour of lost sleep is paid for with one hour of extra sleep. Instead, it can take up to four nights of adequate sleep to make up for one hour lost. In other words, an entire week of insufficient sleep cannot be made up for by sleeping in over a couple of weekend mornings.

Waking during late-morning or early-afternoon hours often results in feeling groggier on arising and difficulties falling asleep the next night. To maximize pressure to sleep, and to improve sleep quality in turn, the key is to avoid naps and aim to keep a consistent wake time daily. For more information on recovering from sleep loss, see Question 5.

## 2. IF YOU ARE HAVING A PROBLEM SLEEPING, YOU AREN'T TRYING HARD ENOUGH TO MONITOR AND FIX IT

Expressions like "pull oneself up by one's bootstraps" reflect the attitude of self-improvement and making personal progress through one's efforts alone, a belief commonly seen in individualistic societies. Those with this belief may suggest that problems sleeping are the result of an individual's lack of willpower to improve the situation. True, sleep problems can result solely from a lack of effort and prioritizing sleep, such as by not consistently making time for at least eight hours of sleep. However, blaming the victim as the cause of the ongoing problem is often unfair and unproductive, and it oversimplifies the situation. Many sources outside our control can result in sleep problems, such as environmental noise, medication changes made by a physician, poor bedding due to financial limitations, seasonal allergies, and so on. In fact, encouraging people to "try harder" to sleep often backfires. If we could simply force ourselves to sleep by willpower alone, then nobody would suffer from insomnia. But people do suffer from insomnia because falling asleep is an involuntary process that cannot be directly controlled. When our efforts to force sleep inevitably fail, our frustration wakes us more. So, the more we try to force sleep, the less likely we are to achieve it. On the other hand, when we try to relax without sleeping (like when watching a movie in the evening), sleep often comes unexpectedly, unfolding naturally following relaxation. Lastly, encouraging others to "monitor" their sleep often increases focus on sleeping problems, causing increased anxiety that itself disrupts sleep. In summary, if you are having problems sleeping, do not try to force sleep but instead find ways to relax. For more information on techniques and strategies for improving sleep and relaxing, see Question 39.

## 3. IT'S IMPORTANT TO REMEMBER AND BE GUIDED BY YOUR DREAMS

In Jewish theology, the Talmud states that "[a]n uninterpreted dream is like throwing away an unopened letter from God." The belief that dreams are meaningful has been shared by many cultures throughout history. Science later reinforced the idea that dreams are a coded message awaiting deciphering when neurologist Sigmund Freud proposed that dream recollection was necessary to resolve emotional problems. Carl Jung later proposed dream interpretation to uncover the hidden meaning of dreams, and many people believe in this even today. But modern research suggests dreams serve other purposes; mainly, they help maintain emotional health, assist in learning and memory, and offer creative solutions to life's challenges. Although some mental health and social benefits may emerge when people journal their dreams or share them with others, surprisingly, some evidence suggests that dreams may actually have no purpose and are simply a side effect of other processes occurring in the brain during particular stages of sleep. The statement that dreams are "important to remember" is also difficult because we cannot fully trust the accuracy of our dream memories. Unlike a video recorder, human memory is highly fallible, suggestible, and easily changed over time. Considering this, dream analysis is somewhat futile when the accuracy of the dream memory is uncertain. Finally, a foundational scientific principle proposed by the philosopher Karl Popper defined a theory as scientific only if research could potentially test and disprove it. The claim that dreams are inherently meaningful messages from the unconscious is an interesting theory, but it is not scientific. This is because there is no way to test this idea or prove that dreams are not a message from the unconscious. For more information on the purpose and meaning of dreams, see Question 10.

## 4. TEENS WHO GO TO BED LATE AND SLEEP IN ARE BEING LAZY

Or, "if you simply went to bed earlier, you wouldn't have such a hard time waking up in the morning." Everyone procrastinates or feels lazy from time to time, but these excuses miss the mark when it comes to teen sleep. Instead, both late bedtimes and late wake times are explained by changes that normally occur during the teenage years. The circadian rhythm is the brain's body clock, which controls the timing of sleep through the release of a brain chemical called melatonin after sunset (i.e., darkness). Just as many older adults are inclined to eat an "early bird" dinner, go to bed in the early evening, and awaken prior to sunrise, teenagers are inclined in the opposite direction. That is, if given the choice and freedom, most teens would go to bed later at night and awaken later the next morning compared to middle-aged adults.

This timing adjustment is expected during adolescence as melatonin shifts to being released later into the night, delaying sleepiness. Similarly, if forced out of bed prior to the natural awakening time, extreme morning grogginess and difficulties in both awakening and remaining awake result. This shift in the timing of sleep and wakefulness is called a delayed sleep phase and is generally not cause for concern during the teenage years. But if it persists long term or interferes with daily functioning (e.g., difficulty arriving to work on time, sleeping through classes, high irritability), it may be classified as a delayed sleep-wake phase disorder. Granted, certain choices and behaviors can make a natural shift become a bigger problem—like late-night studying or socializing, overuse of the "snooze" alarm feature, misuse of caffeine, and use of bright-light electronic devices that further delay melatonin release. For more information on the characteristics of sleep and circadian pressures unique to teenagers, see Question 9.

## 5. IF YOU ARE UNPREPARED FOR A BIG EXAM THE NEXT DAY, IT IS BEST TO STAY UP LATE AND STUDY AS MUCH AS YOU CAN RATHER THAN GET A FULL NIGHT OF SLEEP

It is better to be underprepared but fully rested than underprepared and unrested. The reason people stay up late or "pull an all-nighter" to study before an exam makes sense: *I do not know enough for my exam but every extra hour I spend studying is one more hour of information I can learn for the test.* This reflects a lack of understanding that sleep is critical for memory creation, storage, and recall. To perform well in the exam, the brain must successfully take in new information to short-term memory, move and store it in long-term memory, and later recall information accurately. Sleep is required to effectively move information from short-term to long-term memory. Additionally, when people sleep soon after learning, they are more likely to recall that information—during an exam, for instance—than people who did not sleep. When people sleep fewer than six hours, next day recall is significantly reduced for both previously learned information and new information. Research demonstrates that getting a full night of sleep before an exam will maximize performance. Although it is not possible to learn by listening to audio recordings while sleeping, studying in the evenings may improve later recall. Of course, the best solution would be to study for an exam over an extended period of time, perhaps several weeks, but certainly earlier than the night before. Nevertheless, if one were to find themselves in this position, the better option would be to simply go to bed at a normal time. Maintaining a consistent schedule and sleeping a full eight hours will ensure that the brain can operate at peak performance level during the exam by improving overall recall, thinking speed, and critical thinking. For more information on the impact of sleep on learning and memory, see Question 14.

# QUESTIONS AND ANSWERS

# The Basics of Sleep and Dreaming

## I. What is sleep?

We spend about one-third of our lifespan sleeping—this means the average human sleeps around 25 years in total. But wakefulness in the brain is not a two-sided coin, with the brain being either awake or asleep. Instead, it is more like a sphere with many types, levels, and states of awareness. Consciousness is defined as our level of awareness of things inside ourselves—our thoughts, emotions, and body sensations—and of our environment. On the other hand, unconsciousness is an interruption in this awareness as well as a reduced responsiveness to stimulation. So, sleep can be thought of as one type of unconsciousness.

Sleep is a recurring and reversible state of shifted awareness, sometimes called altered consciousness, that is different from normal wakefulness. While awake, the brain often experiences other types of altered consciousness including "zoning out" or daydreaming, boredom, hypnosis, feeling drunk or "high" from drugs, or states of meditation. Importantly, a significant lack of sleep itself can trigger an altered state of consciousness during the day, including hallucinations and a sense of feeling disconnected from reality.

Complete unconsciousness sometimes occurs following a blow to the head, during a coma, after loss of oxygen to the brain, or after heavy drug or alcohol use ("blacking out"), but this is not the same as sleep. Like other forms of unconsciousness, sleep also involves reduced awareness and responsiveness to our environment (sounds, smells, lights, etc.), although sleep is distinct from complete unconsciousness because sleepers can awaken easily with enough environmental stimulation.

During some periods of sleep, the brain is as active as during wakefulness (i.e., during rapid eye movement or REM sleep), but the state of sleep is distinguished by a reduction in body movement. While sleeping, people may move to turn over or briefly jerk or flex muscles in the arms, legs, face, and elsewhere, and rarely, sleepwalking may occur. Generally, though, compared to wakefulness, sleep involves being relatively motionless. During REM sleep, the body naturally and temporarily loses the ability to move most muscles, which prevents people from acting out their dreams and becoming hurt or waking up.

The unique brain activity of sleep is strikingly different from other types of consciousness. Moving into sleep from wakefulness is less like an on/off light switch, with two distinct states, and more like a dimmer switch with a gradual fade between each state. Sleep itself has multiple states of consciousness or sleep stages, with deep sleep (stage N3) being somewhat more difficult to awaken from than light sleep (stage N1). See Question 2 for more information on sleep stages and brain activity.

Sometimes, the term "sleep" is used in ways that do not refer to actual sleep. For example, veterinarians sometimes use the term sleep to mean death, when the reference is to putting a severely ill pet animal "to sleep." And when doctors use medication to induce a temporary state of unconsciousness prior to surgery, they sometimes refer to this as "going to sleep" to reassure patients who are nervous about anesthesia. These changes in consciousness are not the same as sleep.

In summary, sleep is a recurring and reversible state of shifted awareness and consciousness characterized by unique brain activity, reduced movement, decreased environmental awareness, and the ability to return to wakefulness relatively rapidly.

## 2. What is the sleep cycle, and what are the differences between sleep stages?

Sleep is not a uniform and unchanging state across the entire night. Instead, normal sleep includes a set of stages repeating throughout the night, with each set of stages called a sleep cycle. Over an average night, sleep follows a predictable pattern of four to six complete sleep cycles lasting 90–120 minutes each. People often awaken briefly between complete cycles. This momentary awakening may be due to our ancestors' need to regularly check for predators or threats throughout the night. Healthy sleepers typically return to sleep so rapidly following these awakenings that they have no memory of waking up.

Each complete sleep cycle consists of both rapid eye movement (REM) sleep and non-REM (NREM) sleep. REM sleep is accompanied by richly detailed and story-like dreams, usually associated with the quick darting eye movements from which REM gets its name. The ability to move muscles connected to the skeleton is also lost during REM sleep; this is known as paralysis and most likely serves to prevent wakefulness or injury from acting out dreams.

Body temperature falls to its lowest point of the sleep cycle during REM. Breathing rate, heart rate, and blood pressure all increase and become more variable in this stage. Heart rate and blood pressure changes are responsible for increased genital blood flow (i.e., erections in males and swelling of the clitoris in females) seen in REM, changes that are unrelated to whether dreams contain sexual content.

NREM consists of several sleep stages that gradually transition from wakefulness to sleep onset (stage N1) and then from light sleep (stage N2) to deep sleep (stage N3). The subtlety of these transitions is demonstrated when a sleeper is awakened from stage N1 sleep—about 75 percent of the time the sleeper will report that they were still awake and not yet sleeping. While one can awaken fairly quickly from REM, N1, and N2, people in deep N3 sleep are less responsive to their environment, are harder to awaken, and will be disoriented for a brief period of time after awakening. It is possible to dream during NREM sleep but these dreams tend to be fleeting images or thoughts rather than the detailed stories experienced in REM.

During NREM sleep, there is a decrease in heart rate, blood pressure, breathing, kidney function, and urine production. In addition, breathing and heart rate become more regular during NREM compared to wakefulness. Body temperature drops by 2–3° F and digestion slows as well. Several hormones are created and released by the body during NREM sleep. This includes release of melatonin from the brain's pineal gland to influence and maintain daily cycles of sleep as well as the release of growth hormone in deep sleep to stimulate cell repair and growth throughout the body. Cortisol (the "stress hormone") is released later in the sleep period to aid in awakening.

The primary way in which sleep professionals distinguish sleep stages from one another is by the unique brainwaves that characterize each stage. Brainwaves are a result of differences in the frequency, intensity, and patterns of firing of neurons (the messenger cells of the brain). As we transition from wakefulness to sleep, brainwaves slow down as neurons fire signals in a more coordinated manner (resulting in unique wave patterns called vertex sharp waves). The appearance of brief bursts of unique, fast-frequency brainwaves (called sleep spindles and K complexes) marks the transition into stage N2. During stage N3, also known as slow-wave sleep, slower brainwave frequencies predominate. In REM, sleep brainwaves appear randomly with low-intensity "sawtooth waves" (named for their similarity to jagged saw blades when visualized in sleep studies). REM brainwaves look very much like those of someone who is awake.

In well-rested people, it may take 10–20 minutes to fall asleep at the beginning of the night. During this time, the muscles relax and the eyes begin rolling slowly back and forth. This is followed by light sleep (stage N1) that gradually transitions into stage N2 sleep and sometimes into deep sleep (stage N3). Eventually, this leads into REM sleep before shifting back to either brief wakefulness or light sleep at the end of each cycle.

Over the course of the night, the percentage of time spent in each sleep stage shifts. Generally, deep, slow-wave N3 sleep is most common during the first half of the night and becomes less frequent later in the night. Among children and teens, slow-wave sleep is more intense and frequent compared to adults. While slow-wave sleep is sometimes nearly absent in older adults, it typically occurs in cycles throughout the entire night among children and teenagers. There is a gradual though significant decline in the frequency of slow-wave sleep (about 40 percent) throughout the teenage years and into young adulthood (see Question 8 for more discussion on sleep across the lifespan).

REM sleep takes up approximately 25 percent of the total sleep time, and the remaining time is spent in NREM. REM is very brief during the first half of sleep, but it becomes more frequent and longer in duration during the latter half of the sleep period. Due to the relationship between REM sleep and dreaming, the longer that people sleep, the more likely they are to recall dreams. As discussed in Question 3, the purpose and benefits of each sleep stage vary but each has an important function.

### 3. Why do we need sleep, and is it possible to train your body to sleep less?

All animals sleep, including humans. When prevented from sleeping over a long period of time, animals die. So, sleep is unquestionably necessary for survival. But to thrive, to achieve peak mental, physical, social, and emotional performance, good quality sleep is necessary. There is not a single organ or system in the body that isn't negatively affected by sleep loss. But the reverse is equally true; good quality sleep is the best medicine for achieving and maintaining peak health.

Sleep has many purposes, beginning with healthy brain functioning. The brain works faster when it is well rested, helping us to improve our reaction time and focus, which in turn decreases our risk of accidents. Overall, when we sleep well, our safety improves as mental abilities flourish. Getting enough sleep, particularly REM sleep, increases creativity and our ability to efficiently solve problems during the daytime. Sleep also enables us to think rationally about complex topics and make decisions more effectively.

One of the greatest mental benefits of sleep—especially stages N2 and N3 of NREM—is that it promotes learning and memory. Good quality sleep before learning prepares the brain to absorb more information, while sleep after learning helps to store new information and recall it at a later time. In other words, we will struggle to remember what we learn if we don't get enough sleep the night before, or the night after, learning. Given the amount of new academic, social, and extracurricular information teenagers are exposed to, it is no surprise that the need for sleep is greater among teens in comparison to older adults.

Learning involves building strong connections between neurons, the messenger cells of the brain. But normal brain functioning also creates waste byproducts and extra substances, much like exhaust from a car engine, that build up over time and can become toxic to the brain if not eliminated. Sleep acts like a janitor for the brain, eliminating this waste and unnecessary connections between neurons as well as reinforcing important new connections between neurons to support learning. It is likely that the lack of this "brain janitor" is the cause of death in experiments where rats are experimentally prevented from sleeping over a month. This may also explain why humans who sleep fewer than seven hours on most nights typically die younger than those who sleep more.

In addition to increasing the life span, getting enough sleep provides protection from a variety of dangerous or deadly medical conditions including cancer, obesity, dementia, heart disease, stroke, heart attack, and diabetes. When sleep-deprived, our immune system works less effectively, increasing our chances of catching a cold or flu and decreasing the effectiveness of vaccines.

One way in which sleep promotes physical health is by triggering the secretion of growth hormone from the brain's pituitary gland; this helps repair and build new cells throughout the body. Most teenagers need around nine hours of sleep nightly to obtain the optimal levels of growth hormone needed to support major cell development seen throughout puberty.

This cell growth also explains why sleep is associated with increased muscle strength, speed, and better athletic performance. Aside from the physical benefits of sleep in general, REM sleep helps support psychological and emotional stability. In other words, another purpose of sleep is self-therapy. Without enough sleep, we become more depressed, anxious, irritable, and suspicious and less able to cope with stress.

The inactivity theory of sleep suggests that safety is another purpose of sleep and that safety is enhanced by staying in place. During evolution, sleeping kept humans and primates motionless and quiet, preventing them from wandering through the darkness. This kept them out of harm's way, preventing them from being attacked by nighttime predators. The absence of artificial light prevented early humans from engaging in significant nighttime activity, so sleep may also serve to save energy during the night, which is typically an unproductive time. This theory is supported by findings that the human metabolism slows down by about 10 percent during sleep.

Although sleep is a private experience, it is necessary for successful social functioning. Sufficient REM sleep is related to our ability to read the facial expressions of other people. Given the importance of nonverbal communication in our interactions with others, this skill improves relationships by enhancing understanding and empathy and also makes it easier to detect nonverbal threats. Sleep also helps us appear more attractive to others by increasing blood circulation, building skin collagen (the most common protein in the body, which acts like a glue providing structure to cells), decreasing wrinkles, reducing dark and puffy bags under the eyes, and protecting the skin from sun damage. Question 16 further explores the effect of sleep on relationships.

To maximize the benefits of sleep, infants need 12–17 hours of sleep, children need 9–15 hours, teenagers need 8–10 hours, and adults need at least 7 hours. While it is possible to survive on less sleep than these recommendations, one's quality of life and life span will decrease. There is a genetic variation that allows some people to thrive on only 6 hours of sleep nightly, but this characteristic is extraordinarily rare.

Unfortunately, it is not possible to train your body to sleep less. There are no known instances of someone remaining awake for more than a few days before surrendering to sleep. Some people report that they function well with just four or five hours of sleep nightly, but scientific measurement of their mental, physical, and psychological functioning easily demonstrates that they are not operating at peak performance level. When sleep is deprived over the long term, people lose awareness of how impaired they are in reality. Functioning in a sleep-deprived state begins to feel normal over time because people essentially forget what being fully rested feels like.

When not sleeping enough at night, some people take several, short "power naps" throughout the day to make up for lost sleep. However, napping does not provide most of the benefits earned from nighttime sleep, like improved emotional regulation or cellular building and repair. The only notable benefit to napping is improvement in alertness and concentration, although this effect is temporary.

Caffeine postpones but does not prevent the need for sleep. If a drug were invented that could truly eliminate the need for sleep, it likely would quickly dethrone caffeine from its current title of "world's most popular drug." Given the potential profit that would come from finding such a medicine, pharmaceutical companies have worked tirelessly to find one, but it does not exist. Militaries have also invested millions into research for such a drug to gain advantage on the battlefield, but these efforts have come up short as well. Perhaps the discovery of a drug that eliminates the need for sleep is no more likely than finding a drug that eliminates the need to breathe oxygen. Sleep is so critical for life that such a drug likely cannot exist.

In summary, it is challenging to answer the deceptively simple question "Why do we sleep?" in a concise way because we sleep for many reasons and benefits. But the most basic answer is that we sleep to survive and thrive—in other words, to live long, happy, and healthy lives.

## 4. Why do we get sleepy?

The primary cause of feeling sleepy is what scientists call homeostatic regulation, or more simply, the sleep drive. As cells burn energy throughout the day, a byproduct called adenosine is released into the parts of the brain required for wakefulness. The longer we are awake, the more the adenosine that's built up. In a sense, adenosine is like sleep fuel: the more it accumulates in the brain through the day, the sleepier we feel, the faster we fall asleep, the deeper we sleep (i.e., the larger the amount of slow-wave sleep we have), and the more successful we are at remaining asleep. If this sleep fuel becomes too high over the course of a day, we eventually cannot fight against it and will sleep whether we want to or not—and regardless of safety, such as when driving.

The buildup of adenosine molecules through the day eventually begins to obstruct brain cell activity responsible for wakefulness, especially in the lower front area of the brain known as the basal forebrain. Adenosine specifically increases sleepiness by suppressing the effects of orexin (also known as hypocretin), a small chemical protein that promotes wakefulness throughout the brain. So, when we are "fighting" to stay awake, we are struggling against adenosine buildup and the natural drive to sleep.

Assuming you have been getting enough sleep most nights, when you wake up in the morning there is very little adenosine buildup in your brain. But as the day progresses, this sleep fuel increases steadily with every passing minute and with it, feelings of sleepiness gradually increase. Acting like the brain's stopwatch, adenosine tracks how long we've been awake. During sleep, adenosine is cleared from the brain. A full night of sleep provides enough time to eliminate all the adenosine sleep fuel and helps us wake up feeling refreshed. But insufficient sleep results in a person feeling sleepy on awakening because not all the adenosine was eliminated.

As discussed in Question 37, caffeine temporarily decreases sleepiness by partly blocking brain receptors for adenosine for up to 16 hours, thereby delaying the pressure to sleep and enhancing feelings of wakefulness. Caffeine acts like a blindfold, preventing the brain from knowing how much adenosine is already present and that it is continually rising. However, this blindfold begins to come off around five to eight hours after caffeine consumption, once it begins to be cleared from the body. This sometimes results in an experience called a "caffeine crash" as adenosine brain receptors—previously blocked by caffeine—become rapidly overwhelmed by the incoming rush of backlogged adenosine that had been building outside awareness.

While recent scientific advances have revealed the different roles of other brain chemicals (neurotransmitters) on sleep and wakefulness, we do not yet fully understand these complex interactions. Like adenosine, GABA is another sleep-promoting brain substance that switches off the brain's arousal centers. Another chemical called serotonin is also used by the brain to create melatonin, which promotes sleep. For more information on causes of sleepiness and fatigue, see Question 21.

### 5. If I skip a night of sleep or "pull an all-nighter," how long does it take to "catch up" on lost sleep?

Lost sleep is forever lost. What this means is the negative impact of skipping a night of sleep cannot really be completely undone. When we fail to meet our sleep need—which for teens usually falls between 8 and 10 hours—we build up a "sleep debt." Pulling an all-nighter and remaining awake for more than 24 hours creates a significant debt, and this debt is paid back with interest (which is to say, we don't pay back one hour of lost sleep with just one extra hour of sleep). More precisely, some research suggests it can take four nights of adequate sleep to make up for only one hour of sleep debt. While it is possible to "catch up" by sleeping longer than normal on nights following lost sleep, it can take up to 14 days of oversleeping to compensate for a single all-nighter.

The body and brain are very resilient and even if we were to remain awake for several nights, or even for a week, we are unlikely to die as long as we avoid operating motor vehicles or heavy machinery. Sleep-deprived people are much more impaired than they might appreciate, which can have deadly consequences. After 16 hours of wakefulness, brain performance begins to suffer across the board and mental abilities rapidly decline. After remaining awake all night, the brain will attempt to achieve sleep in small chunks, called microsleeps, that last several seconds. To the outside observer, the person may appear awake with eyes open, but their brain is technically asleep with a temporary loss of awareness of the outside world. The consequences of these brief lapses in concentration while driving at high speeds can be lethal.

After remaining awake one night, a person struggles to maintain attention. But even after three nights of full recovery sleep, concentration will still remain poorer than normal. In other words, catching up on lost sleep over a two-day weekend is not enough to recover from shortfalls in attention and concentration. Short naps of 20–30 minutes, or consuming caffeine, may provide a temporary improvement in concentration, but naps do nothing to address problems in physical and mental health following sleep loss.

The day following an all-nighter, it is much harder to learn and the new information will be forgotten more rapidly; recall of information in general is also more difficult. Research conducted with rats shows that even a single night of sleep deprivation causes negative effects on the activity of learning-related genes in the brain's memory center (hippocampus).

To use a practical human example, if someone stays awake all night to cram for a morning exam, their performance on the exam is likely to be worse than what it would be if they had gone to bed the night before at a reasonable hour. Additionally, any new information taught in afternoon classes following the exam would be more difficult to learn. Even following two full nights of recovery sleep, the person will recall 40 percent less information from the afternoon classes than if they had not pulled an all-nighter earlier; also, the remaining 60 percent of learned information will be forgotten more rapidly.

On recovery nights following total sleep deprivation, if allowed to sleep as long as possible, most adults will sleep an average of 10–12 hours, and teens may sleep longer. Recovering sleep initially includes more NREM sleep than normal, during which the body works overtime to remove excess adenosine—the chemical responsible for sleepiness—from the body. But on subsequent nights, people will spend significantly more time in REM and enter into the first REM stage of the night more rapidly than normal, an experience known as REM rebound.

Unfortunately, napping or sleeping in on the weekend is unlikely to significantly reduce sleep debt, and these can interfere with our sleep cycle and body clock in other ways. For example, napping might provide short-term relief from sleepiness by reducing adenosine, but like snacking before a meal, it may make the body less "hungry" for sleep at bedtime because naps reduce the nighttime sleep drive. Sleeping in too late into the day in an attempt to recover lost sleep can sometimes backfire as well. When oversleeping and awakening during late-morning or early-afternoon hours, around the time when the body naturally experiences a dip in energy, people sometimes report feeling groggier on awakening.

Other unhelpful strategies some use to "hack" sleep or beat the system are: sleeping in several chunks throughout the day and night; sleeping the same number of hours over a period of days while varying the timing of sleep from one day to the next; and "banking" or saving up sleep in advance of an all-nighter. But because these interfere with the regularity of sleep, they are all ultimately unhelpful, unhealthy, and unwise.

In summary, for the best quality of sleep—and to achieve the peak mental, physical, and psychological performance that it enables—the most important factors are consistent and sufficient sleep. For teens, this means sleeping 8–10 hours in one unified period and around the same time every night. The body clock that regulates alertness throughout the day and night (circadian rhythm) is strongest when we keep a consistent routine. The sleep drive (homeostatic process) that helps us fall and remain asleep works most effectively when we avoid napping and keep a regular bedtime and wake time. So, pulling all-nighters—or any other behavior that interferes with this regularity—negatively impacts our sleep and overall health in ways that can last up to several weeks.

## 6. What is the ideal sleep environment?

The best sleep environment can be determined by reflecting on the evolution of sleep in primates to meet their needs for safety and conservation of body energy. Specifically considering our Neanderthal "caveman" ancestors, our brains inherited a preference to sleep in a cave-like environment. To put it simply, individuals sleep best when their surroundings are dark, quiet, cool, and safe.

When sleeping inside a cave or outside under the stars, our ancestors may have been surrounded by darkness or, perhaps, the warm amber glow of campfires. However, at night, they would have experienced only dim light and no light in the blue range of the light spectrum. Blue spectrum light is the wavelength abundant in sunlight that suppresses the brain chemical melatonin and helps maintain wakefulness during the day. In modern times, since darkness is best for sleep, humans need to be especially careful to avoid nighttime blue light exposure, which, in addition to daylight, is commonly associated with light emitting diode (LED) light bulbs and backlit screens such as computers, phones, and televisions. These LED devices can trick the brain into thinking the sun is still up, keeping our body clock (circadian rhythm) on alert and preventing sleep. Even when the eyes are closed, light can be detected to some degree through the eyelids and may negatively impact sleep quality. In situations where light exposure cannot be controlled (e.g., streetlights, roommates using LED screens, etc.), individuals benefit from the use of an eye mask or blackout curtains.

When sleeping outdoors, our ancestors likely had to awaken regularly to check for predators, maintain the fire, and ensure safety. Safety is less of a concern in the modern world where we mostly sleep behind locked doors. But places and situations that feel different or unsafe (e.g., hotels, dangerous neighborhoods, camping) may disrupt sleep quality, particularly on the first night in a new environment. Finally, loud or inconsistent noises—such as traffic, television commercials, or construction—can disrupt sleep. Earplugs can mask noises effectively and improve sleep quality; "white noise" devices that mask other noises (e.g., a white noise machine, a loud fan, phone apps) also do the same.

Our bodies have adapted to sleeping outdoors, and therefore we sleep best when the environment is cool. As we fall asleep, our body temperature drops; this helps us sleep more deeply, with the best quality sleep occurring at 65°F (18.3°C). In addition to adjusting the thermostat, it's a good idea to consider the use of a bedroom fan and avoid excessive bedding that can cause overheating.

For teenagers, sleep position doesn't matter much, and they can sleep in whatever way feels most comfortable. But as we get older, medical issues may direct the sleep position that is best for us. Sleeping on the back is best for low back and hip pain and to avoid wrinkles, but this can worsen neck pain and sleep-related breathing disorders like sleep apnea and snoring. A special pillow to cradle the neck may help shoulder or neck pain while a pillow beneath the knees can sometimes reduce back pain.

Sleeping on the stomach may help with breathing difficulties, but this is also associated with acne breakouts common in teens. A wedge pillow that keeps the upper body elevated on an incline may reduce mild snoring. Sleeping on the right side can worsen heartburn and acid reflux, but these improve when sleeping on the left side. Sleeping on either side, particularly in the fetal position or with a pillow between your knees, is best during pregnancy, aids digestion, and may reduce snoring. However, side sleeping can be associated with jaw pain or tightness.

It is a good idea to regularly replace pillows, bedding, and old mattresses as they wear out or become soiled. While pillows and mattresses should provide support, very expensive specialty bedding options are often unnecessary. Softness or firmness should be based on your personal preference. Regularly cleaning bedding can also reduce breathing problems during sleep resulting from dust and other allergy-causing substances.

## 7. Is it true that people in the past got much more sleep than we do today?

The technology necessary to scientifically measure sleep did not exist until the 20th century, so accounts of sleep length prior to this time are based on self-report, such as those found in personal journal entries. Despite this limitation, historians have investigated sleep throughout history and concluded that while it is true that people slept differently in the past, they probably did not sleep more than we do today.

Prior to the invention of the light bulb in the 1800s, the timing of human activity and sleep was largely dictated by sunlight. Within a few hours after sundown, humans would begin the first of two phases of nighttime sleep, also known as biphasic sleep. After three to five hours of sleep and around the middle of the night—literally where the word "midnight" gets its name—people would awaken for several hours. This was followed by them returning to sleep for another three to four hours and awakening with the sunrise.

During these midnight awakenings lasting one to two hours, people would do a variety of activities such as dream interpretation, prayer, taking medicine, and checking to ensure safety. Some physicians of the day believed that sex after the first sleep interval was more enjoyable and more likely to result in pregnancy.

Some historians have identified a variation of this biphasic sleep in other cultures, where people obtained roughly seven hours of nighttime sleep and an additional afternoon nap of one to two hours. This nap is the forerunner of the midday sleep called the "siesta" which is practiced even today in many cultures, particularly in warmer climates.

After the light bulb became commonplace and modern sleepers moved to a single phase of sleep, the middle of the sleep period shifted from midnight for most people to 2:45 a.m. for adults and 3:50 a.m. for teenagers. The shift toward a single sleep period was also reinforced by the societal adoption of the eight-hour workweek during the Industrial Revolution (the eight-hour workweek was originally proposed by Welsh socialist Robert Owen who argued for "eight hours labor, eight hours recreation, eight hours rest" in 1817).

In summary, the modern sleep length of between seven and nine hours in adults is essentially the same as the sleep length of early humans, with only a difference in timing. It can be argued that the modern desire to achieve a full eight to nine hours of uninterrupted nighttime sleep, without even brief awakenings, is unrealistic. These worries about achieving perfect sleep may, ironically, cause anxiety and alertness that in turn create problems sleeping.

## 8. How does sleep change over a lifetime?

Imagine a quiet home inhabited by a large family at 4:00 a.m. A newborn baby is sleeping in a crib a few feet away from his parents; another room is being shared by his teenage sister and his five-year-old sister; in yet another bedroom are his elderly grandparents. All of them may be asleep at 4:00 a.m., but all are likely in different sleep stages with highly varied depth and quality.

Sleep patterns change a great deal across a person's lifespan due to normal maturation of the brain, aging, and the demands of daily life. The greatest changes in sleep occur across a baby's first year of life. The newborn is likely to be sleeping between 17 and 18 hours daily and waking every two or three hours to be fed or comforted. Much to the frustration of their sleep-deprived parents, until six months of age (or even afterward), babies' brains do not have a fully developed body clock, called the circadian rhythm. This system synchronizes sleep to regular cycles of day and night. As the brain matures and day-to-day activities—such as feeding schedule and indoor light exposure—become more regular, a baby's sleep eventually begins to occur primarily during the night. However, even at the age of one year, many babies will wake up one or more times a night.

The brainwaves of sleeping newborns look quite different from those of adults. Although adults spend around 20 percent of their sleep time in REM, a newborn spends about half of its sleep time in a REM-like period called active sleep. Unlike adult REM, active sleep involves small movements of the mouth, limbs, or fingers and likely takes up a greater portion of the night because this type of sleep accelerates brain development. When there is so much to be learned and remembered in the baby's new world, active sleep promotes learning through the formation of new connections between brain cells. The other half of a baby's sleep is a period of stillness called quiet sleep.

By the end of their first year of life, babies' sleep brainwaves begin to resemble those of adults. Quiet sleep begins to occupy a greater portion of nightly sleep and evolves into three distinguishable NREM stages, while active sleep comes to resemble adult REM sleep (see Question 2 for more information about sleep stages). When babies have difficulty getting to sleep, it may be due to teething or illness or because the baby is overstimulated. It may also be due to normal separation anxiety, as babies of certain ages will sometimes not go to sleep unless a familiar caretaker is nearby.

Many cultural beliefs and practices influence how babies sleep. These include whether and for how long babies are nursed, feelings with regard to whether babies should sleep in the same bed or bedroom as parents, and attitudes concerning whether babies need intentional training by caregivers to "learn" how to sleep through the night. Although these things do not appear to affect babies' total number of hours of sleep, they influence the pattern and rhythm of the babies' sleep throughout the day and night.

In early childhood, NREM sleep is primarily marked by deeper slow-wave sleep than in adults, and across later childhood, the portion of sleep spent in REM gradually decreases. About 40 percent of children have some kind of sleep problem, although they often grow out of it. Most children have an occasional bad dream, especially during ages when fear of the dark or of monsters is common. Other sleep problems may occur when a child is ill or dealing with change, like starting a new school or family tensions. Other typical problems include refusing to go to bed, sleepwalking, and having difficulty falling and staying asleep. There is increasing concern that preschool and school-age children aren't getting enough sleep because drinking beverages containing caffeine and using electronic devices has become more common among them in recent decades.

Puberty activates a biological delay in daily circadian rhythms, leading teens to favor later bedtimes and wake times. The brain chemical melatonin, which assists in falling asleep, builds up later in the evening during adolescence. This delays feelings of sleepiness until later in the night. Academic, extracurricular, and work obligations, as well as late-night social events, also delay bedtimes. Compared to the rest of the population, more teens and young adults would describe themselves as "night owls"—people who find they think and function better in the late evening compared to the morning. Although these changes are a normal part of puberty, early waking times demanded by school or work can further massively disrupt sleep and daily functioning. See Question 9 for more on delayed sleep during adolescence and Question 18 for common sleep disorders during adolescence.

Adulthood is associated with changes in both homeostatic sleep drive (how much sleep we get) and circadian rhythm (how regularly we sleep). Total sleep need decreases slightly, from 8 to 10 hours during adolescence to 7–9 hours during adulthood. For reasons we do not fully understand, circadian rhythms continue to shift throughout adulthood to earlier timing preferences. While teenagers commonly have later bedtimes and wake times, older adults are likely to feel sleepy earlier in the evening and they often wake up early—so they are often called "morning larks." Compared to younger people, older adults also obtain less deep sleep each night. They are more likely to take daytime naps, wake up after falling asleep, and remain awake during the night. Medical conditions common in older adults, such as pain or needing to use the bathroom, as well as the medications prescribed to manage them may further disrupt sleep.

Returning to the home described earlier, we can confidently assume that the family members' sleep will vary greatly due to differences in sleep stages, homeostatic sleep pressure, and circadian rhythms. At 4:00 a.m., the teenager might be in the middle of her nightly sleep cycle and very possibly in deep, slow-wave sleep. As the infant squirms and prepares for a middle-of-the-night feeding, his adult caregiver transitions into lighter sleep overall, interspersed with periods of REM and wakefulness as the baby's needs dictate. Meanwhile, with their bodies' release of alerting hormones like cortisol, the grandparents are preparing to wake up for the day.

### 9. I can't get to sleep before midnight, and then I like to sleep until late in the morning—isn't that normal for teenagers?

It is common for teenagers to have late bedtimes and wake times. This relates primarily to normal circadian rhythm changes following puberty as well as to lifestyle and the homeostatic sleep drive. Circadian rhythm is a term used for the regular daily biological cycles of the body. It is responsible for the timing of sleep and wakefulness, changes in body temperature, release of hormones, digestion, and other physical functions. The circadian rhythm is controlled by an area deep in the brain called the suprachiasmatic nucleus, our central timekeeper. This body clock influences when we feel sleepy and when we want to wake up using cues from the environment to track the passage of time. These cues are called "zeitgebers," a German word meaning "time giver."

The timing of light exposure and its frequency or color (i.e., white and blue spectrum light) is the primary zeitgeber, although environmental temperature and the timing of our daily activities (e.g., meals, exercise, and socializing) also alter daily sleep and wake cycles. In response to zeitgebers, our central timekeeper influences the release of various brain chemicals that keep us awake and alert when necessary. Changes in the levels of these brain chemicals, which include norepinephrine, dopamine, serotonin, histamine, and acetylcholine, can suppress sleep and increase wakefulness. Zeitgebers can also trigger release of the hormone melatonin (primarily during darkness or in the absence of blue spectrum light). Melatonin creates feelings of sleepiness near our usual bedtime and through the sleep period, but it stops being released as the morning approaches to help us awaken.

A person's age and their unique biological characteristics affect the timing of melatonin release in the brain, influencing when they go to sleep and wake up. For reasons that are not fully understood, the nightly release of melatonin shifts across puberty to occur later in the evening. This shift naturally delays the preferred bedtimes of teens and makes it more difficult for them to wake up early. The delay in the evening release of melatonin peaks at around age 20 and can happen as much as two hours later than it does among younger and older people (also see Question 8 on changes in sleep across the life span).

So, for example, a teen who normally went to bed at 10:00 p.m. during childhood may not feel sleepy until midnight. Likewise, a previous preference to wake up around 7:00 a.m. may change during the teenage years to a natural preference to awaken at 9:00 a.m. The problem is that this is often at odds with school start times selected by school administrators, who prefer that students arrive at 8:00 a.m. or earlier because this aligns well with their adult circadian preference. Going to sleep after midnight and waking at 6:00 or 7:00 a.m. for school puts a teen in a chronic state of sleepiness. The Center for Disease Control reported in 2015 that three-quarters of U.S. high school students do not get the recommended minimum eight hours of sleep. Teens often reach for coffee or energy drinks with caffeine to compensate, but this short-term fix and long-term sleep deprivation lead to problems in physical and mental health.

Across the world, many school districts have instituted later school start times supported by research showing that even a one-hour delay in high school start times leads to more sleep, better attendance, less lateness, better mood, improved grades, and even a reduction in teen motor vehicle incidents. In 2022, California became the first U.S. state to act on this research and change school start time to 8:30 a.m. across public schools. But other school districts are reluctant to change start times, arguing that the later work hours inconvenience staff and conflict with afterschool activities like sports, extracurriculars, and jobs.

Preferred bedtime is also influenced by late-night studying, social events, and use of electronic devices with lighted screens, all of which signal "daylight" to the central body clock, suppress evening melatonin release, and postpone sleepiness. Aside from the normal teenage changes in sleep, delayed sleep-wake phase disorder (DSWPD) may be diagnosed if daily functioning is severely impaired due to always being out of sync with the timing and alertness demands of school, work, and social life.

People with DSWPD are often described as "night owls" because they are not sleepy at conventional times but feel more alert and productive late in the evening and night. More common among adolescents and young adults, some believe that DSWPD is an extreme form of the normal changes in bedtime seen in most teens. When present, DSWPD can be treated by maintaining consistent sleep times, using light exposure therapy, advancing bedtime by one hour a night until the desired bedtime is reached, and taking medication. For an example of DSWPD in teens, see Case Study 2, "Up All Night with Nemesis Dawn." Additionally, see Question 18 for more on common sleep disorders among teens.

## 10. Why do we dream?

The purpose and meaning of dreams have fascinated humans throughout recorded history and are still hotly debated today. Many early civilizations believed dreams had religious or personal significance. But modern neuroscience is slowly beginning to reveal the purpose of dreaming, with various studies suggesting dreams may be critical for emotional regulation, problem-solving, memory formation or removal, and mental processing of information.

Dream interpretation was practiced as far back as 2100 BCE by the Sumerians in ancient Mesopotamia, by ancient Egyptians, and by Greek philosophers, many of whom believed dreams were a message from the gods. Formal study of dreams has been recorded by scholars, such as the Islamic philosopher Abu Nasr Al-Farabi during the Middle Ages and Chinese scholar Chen Shiyuan during the 16th century. Much later, Austrian neurologist Sigmund Freud and Swiss psychiatrist Carl Jung came to believe that dream interpretation was useful to successfully resolve emotional problems, a belief that persisted for nearly the entire 20th century.

However, modern science in the 21st century is only just beginning to answer *why* we dream. Dreams typically last from 5 to 20 minutes, and we spend up to two hours nightly in dream sleep. Dreams are recalled about 80 percent of the time when people are awakened from REM sleep: these dreams are usually detailed and story-like and sometimes surreal or emotionally intense. A major barrier to dream research is that there is no way to read the mind of the dreamer (yet); that is, there is no way to directly observe and measure dreams. But analysis of dream self-reports, which are typically gathered by awakening sleepers who are in the REM stage of sleep, have shown that the previous two days of waking-life experience make up the majority of dream content.

Research has already supported the idea that REM sleep helps maintain psychological health and emotional stability, without which we become depressed, anxious, irritable, and stressed. Our social interactions also improve from REM sleep, as we become better able to read nonverbal emotional cues and facial expressions of others the following day. Everyone dreams during REM, whether or not the dreams are recalled the next day, and the benefits of REM sleep (or of dreaming) are present even in the absence of dream recall.

Some argue that the benefits of REM may not necessarily be a direct result of dreaming or that dreaming may just be a byproduct of sleep with no unique purpose or meaning. Interestingly, when people are prevented from entering REM sleep (i.e., by experimentally awakening them every time they enter this stage or by using medications for which suppression of REM is a side effect), no detectable problems in behavior, memory, or emotional stability arise, even over many years. This is dramatically different from the severe negative impact of NREM sleep deprivation. As a result, some scientists conclude that either dreams and REM sleep have no direct function or the benefits they bring are not critical for survival or day-to-day functioning.

Separate from the documented benefits of REM sleep, there is no scientific agreement currently on the unique purpose of REM sleep and dreaming. But recent research using brain scanning machines most strongly supports the idea that the likely purpose of REM dreaming is to maintain strong mental health, to aid creative problem-solving, and to facilitate learning and memory, particularly of personal and emotionally important information.

REM dreams may likely help regulate our mood by removing painful emotional content from memories of the previous day. Some scientists suggest that dreams create stories, which allow us to rehearse feelings and experience emotional responses to imagined narratives and possible life scenarios. This is supported by findings that up to half of our present-day emotional concerns and themes arise during REM dreams. The majority (65 percent) of dreams involve negative emotions like anger, sadness, or fear, while 20 percent include positive emotions like excitement or happiness. Notably, sexual dreams are not very common, occurring in less than 10 percent of all dreams. Promising studies have suggested that REM dreams play a role in recovering from emotional trauma by transforming fearful memories into less threatening thoughts.

Dreams likely also play a role in memory, particularly emotional memory processing, helping us sort through, make sense of, and learn from the positive and negative emotional events of the day. Occasional replaying of past experiences in REM dreams, especially of emotionally charged memories, may also help us gain insight into unanticipated connections between our past and current life circumstances. During REM, the brain's prefrontal cortex or logic center is deactivated, which facilitates creative thinking in dreaming that helps us solve problems relating to life's challenges, discover big-picture links between distant memories or patterns we may not have previously noticed, and come up with creative insights.

In REM, individual memories are also blended together in creative and sometimes strange ways. When trying to make sense of this random noise and imagery, dream content can seem odd and unexplainable, such as when someone recalls that they saw a flock of birds and a woman walking a dog the previous day and subsequently had a dream about a flying dog. Dreams may also connect new emotional information to past personal experiences (autobiographical memory) to strengthen connections, integrating memories from earlier in life in the process. That is, dreams might increase insight, creativity, and our ability to efficiently solve problems during the daytime.

NREM sleep is known to be critical for memory and learning, and dreams can also occur in NREM—although these dreams have less story-like content, resembling something like a fleeting thought while awake. Learning occurs by the building of stronger connections between brain cells (neurons). NREM sleep increases learning by reinforcing new memories and by eliminating unnecessary cellular connections. A side effect of this cleaning process may be dreaming.

As the brain sorts through information from the previous day to determine which connections to discard and which ones to keep, random mental imagery and sensory experiences arise. This is the most likely cause of NREM dreams. Some research suggests dreams that replay memories from the day during NREM help us uncover rules we were previously unaware of, like an epiphany or "aha" moment. In other words, we dream to remember (new information) and to forget (negative emotions and unnecessary connections between neurons).

One major theory describes the role of dreams in transferring information from the brain's short-term memory center, known as the hippocampus (sort of like the cache or Random Access Memory—RAM—in a computer), to the long-term memory center called the neocortex (like the hard disk drive of a computer). While research demonstrates that memories are strengthened and information recall is improved during sleep, debate continues regarding whether dreams themselves play a direct role in this process or are an unintentional side effect of the brain attempting to make sense of the random daily imagery by creating a story based on the dreamer's thoughts, emotions, and experiences.

In summary, why we dream is still up for debate. It is very likely that dreams serve multiple purposes, some of which we do not yet fully understand. While dreams undoubtedly can have personal significance to the dreamer, reflecting their current and past memories, emotions, experiences, thoughts, and personality, it is possible that dreams are simultaneously both entirely meaningful and meaningless. However, the scientific evidence most strongly suggests that dreams are important for maintaining emotional health, learning, and memory and to creatively resolve life's challenges.

## 11. Can you learn to influence or control your dreams?

Although dreaming often feels like a passive viewing experience—something you witness rather than something you can intentionally manage—dreams are in fact controllable, both directly and indirectly. Historically, people struggled to understand the source of dreams and many suggested that diet and food may influence dreams. For example, in the book *The Christmas Carol*, when confronted by the ghost of his old business partner, Ebenezer Scrooge concludes he must be experiencing a bad dream resulting from ". . . an undigested bit of beef, a blot of mustard, a crumb of cheese, a fragment of underdone potato. There's more of gravy than of grave about you, whatever you are!"

While Scrooge may be disappointed to learn that diet has minimal effect on what and how we dream, our daytime behaviors exert more control over our sleep and dreaming than one might expect. More likely than diet to influence dreaming is drinking alcohol, using nicotine or other recreational drugs, and afternoon caffeine use, all of which have been found to disrupt normal dream sleep patterns, decreasing dream frequency or triggering nightmares. Likewise, some prescribed antidepressant medications decrease dream frequency whereas other medications, including some over-the-counter medicines (like melatonin), increase dream frequency and vividness. Disorders that disrupt normal sleep, such as sleep-related breathing disorders, can also cause nightmares.

Bad dreams and nightmares awaken the sleeper, delay returning to sleep due to high stress, and may result in the person eventually avoiding sleep altogether to avoid the dreams. However, this causes sleep deprivation, which in turn is a big risk factor for nightmares. This vicious cycle is further reinforced by stress, as nightmares increase stress but also result from it. In other words, good quality sleep and dreams come to those who follow good stress management and do not ignore their personal mental health needs. Clinical treatments, such as imagery rehearsal therapy for nightmares, and techniques to address underlying problems that indirectly influence dreaming are explored further in Question 44.

One of the most direct ways to influence and control dreams is via lucid dreaming, which is a skill that can be learned but occurs naturally in certain individuals. In fact, frequent lucid dreamers are used in some dream research studies to provide real-time feedback to researchers on what they are visualizing in their dreams using eye or muscle movements to convey Morse code. However, lucid dreaming has not been thoroughly researched and, therefore, is not normally used in clinical treatment.

Lucid dreaming occurs when the sleeper gains awareness that they are experiencing a dream while remaining asleep. Lucid dreaming is most common in childhood and lucidity is often achieved at the end of a nightmare, right before awakening (for example, "No matter how fast I ran from the monster, it felt like my body wasn't moving at all. It just didn't make logical sense, and that's when I realized I was having a nightmare. Then I woke up."). However, some individuals are able to remain asleep and use this sleep insight to begin actively controlling the content of the dream itself. Some small studies have found evidence to support the treatment of nightmares or unwanted dreams by training individuals to control their dreams using lucid dreaming techniques.

To lucid dream, and potentially have the ability to control dream content, two strategies are most often used in studies: mnemonic induction of lucid dreams (MILD) and wake-initiated lucid dreaming (WILD). The primary steps of the MILD technique include first spending about 10 minutes prior to bedtime imagining yourself lucid dreaming, thinking about what type of dream experience you'd like to have. Some practitioners additionally recommend keeping a dream journal to document your dreams from previous nights, which may also help prime the mind to be more "on alert" for dreams and, it is hoped, more likely to "catch" a dream while it is occurring and gain lucid awareness.

Next, pledge to yourself before going to bed that you plan to awaken periodically throughout the night, naturally, and intentionally recall dreams. After reviewing your dreams during these awakenings, verbalize aloud (but quietly, if you have a bed partner) your commitment to lucid dream after returning to sleep. Finally, visualize yourself lucid dreaming as you drift back to sleep.

As discussed in Question 2, we know vivid dreams are most likely to occur in REM sleep, and REM sleep occurs most often—and with longer duration—in the last portion of the night. Therefore, lucid dreaming in REM sleep is most likely to occur in the last few hours before the final awakening. The WILD technique, sometimes referred to as the *wake-back-to-bed* technique, takes advantage of this fact and in so doing increases the odds of lucid dreaming.

Specifically, people following a WILD approach are instructed to set an alarm for one hour earlier than the normal, desired wake time. Once awakened by the alarm, the goal is to remain awake but relaxed for the full hour, imagining the type of lucid dream desired. Much like MILD, state aloud to yourself your commitment to lucid dream and then visualize yourself lucid dreaming as you drift back to sleep. Perhaps because additional steps are added, the WILD technique is generally more effective than MILD used alone.

A third approach, which can be used in combination with the above strategies, is reality testing. This technique works to develop a habit of self-reflection that, it is hoped, carries over into dream sleep. Specifically, people are told to ask themselves at regular times throughout the day, "Am I dreaming right now?" With time, this habit can introduce suspicion into dreams, helping dreamers reflect on whether they might be dreaming. This helps reveal dreams in the moment, offering the dreamer clarity (or lucidity) on their circumstances.

Importantly, none of these lucid dreaming strategies should be used by those with, or at risk for, serious mental health problems like delusions, psychosis, difficulties with reality testing, or paranoia because they could make these difficulties worse. On the other hand, a small 2020 study revealed that lucid dreaming may decrease symptoms of insomnia, anxiety, and depression. So, while scientific support for the clinical use of lucid dreaming is promising though limited, more studies are necessary to fully understand and support the use of lucid dreaming in those with mental health problems.

While it remains to be seen where the science of lucid dreaming will lead, modern sleep research has focused primarily on controlling dreams or nightmares through imagery techniques, cognitive behavioral therapy (CBT) strategies, or use of medicines. These techniques for controlling dreams are explored in greater detail in Question 44.

# The Connection between Sleep, Health, and Performance

## 12. How do sleep and physical health interact?

Each night, sleep helps to restore, repair, and maintain essential body functions so that we can live, be healthy, and thrive the next day. After a good night's sleep, you are more likely to feel energized and to be active and highly involved with friends, family, and others at school and work. All body systems benefit from regular sleep, including the heart and circulatory system, the digestive system, and the immune system. We cannot survive without sleep.

Everyone occasionally has a night of bad sleep, which can lead to grogginess, grumpiness, and a desire to return to bed. People vary with regard to how much they notice the impact of one night of sleep loss. Sometimes energy drinks or caffeine can help us forget a sleepless night, but the body keeps track. For example, a night of less than six hours of sleep (or even just two or three hours less than one's regular sleep time) can produce measurable problems with alertness—you may find it harder to think creatively, solve problems, and multitask. Sleep deprivation additionally increases the likelihood of accidents or injury.

During sleep, the body produces new cells to replace the ones damaged by daily exposure to stress, physical activity, and ultraviolet rays.

The hormone melatonin, which helps regulate our day-night sleep cycles, also suppresses the growth of tumors and may protect against cancer. In addition, the defense cells of the immune system (e.g., T cells, cytokines) flourish during sleep, helping to protect the body from viruses, infections, and other risks. When people don't get at least eight hours of sleep, the body is less effective in defending against colds and other infections, and toxic substances that are normally cleared from the brain during sleep are not fully eliminated.

"Lose weight while you sleep" may sound too good to be true, but people who sleep fewer than six hours per night are more likely to be overweight. Research shows that inadequate sleep increases levels of the hormone ghrelin, which intensifies cravings for high-fat, high-carbohydrate food (like junk food), and decreases leptin, a hormone responsible for feeling full. In combination, as people crave less-healthy food more often and don't feel full after eating, weight increases. In other words, an important part of any weight loss or weight maintenance plan should include prioritizing sleep.

Although not always noticeable, insufficient sleep over time may cause the heart to work harder, resulting in high blood pressure. Acknowledging the importance of sleep on heart health, the American Heart Association, in 2022, added sleep to its "Life's Essential 8" recommendations. In addition to recognizing sleep as an essential lifestyle and health factor that helps maintain the circulatory system and prevents heart disease, the Life's Essential 8 also emphasize maintaining a healthy diet, daily physical activity levels, avoiding cigarette smoke exposure, and maintaining normal body mass, balanced blood sugar, and low blood cholesterol levels. Notably, following long-term insufficient sleep, increased levels of blood cholesterol circulate, contributing to hardening of the arteries. This makes it more difficult for blood to flow freely through the circulatory system, which increases risk for heart attack and stroke (i.e., blockage and breakage of arteries).

Given the genetic risks for certain diseases, as well as the link between sleep and physical health, undoubtedly those with a family history of chronic illness would benefit from prioritizing sleep earlier in life. Not getting enough sleep reduces the body's response to insulin, the hormone that helps the body use the sugar we eat for our energy needs. In the long run, this increases risk of developing diabetes. Maintaining healthy sleep habits and aiming for at least eight hours of sleep nightly is a critical part of preventing high blood pressure or heart disease in someone who has family members with the same condition.

In sum, regular and sufficient sleep is one of the greatest gifts teens can give themselves. Along with good nutrition, exercise, sunlight, and supportive friends, good sleep is your investment toward your best days and a longer and happier future.

## 13. How does sleep influence athletic performance?

When Coach told you to practice for the big game, you were probably thinking you should drill down on your free throws or do some extra goal kicks. Getting to sleep early might have been the last thing on your mind . . . but arguably, sleep was the most important "practice" you could get.

In addition to the general physical benefits of sleep discussed in Question 12, getting at least eight hours of sleep is necessary for peak endurance, strength, decision-making, speed, and athletic success. Sleep supports the release of growth hormone from the brain's pituitary gland, which helps the body repair muscles after heavy workouts. This may also lead to better energy levels and training quality. Sleep balances cortisol release from the adrenal glands, which helps to manage the physical and mental stress of training and competition. During sleep, the body produces cytokines and T cells, supporting the immune response to infection and reducing the likelihood and severity of illness. Research has also shown that athletes are less likely to get injured on days when they have received more sleep the night before.

Almost every measure of athletic performance benefits from good sleep. In a 2011 study, college basketball players were encouraged to try to increase their regular sleep to 10 hours nightly for around six weeks. The results were astonishing: the athletes improved in shooting accuracy, they ran faster, and they reported reduced sleepiness and overall well-being. Similar results have been found for tennis and soccer players and for swimmers. When those athletes improved their sleep hygiene practices and increased their nightly sleep, they showed improved coordination, reaction time, and kick strength as well as reduced daytime fatigue.

However, not getting enough sleep reverses these benefits. In addition to worsening stamina, concentration, and coordination, a lack of sleep changes how the body ingests and uses food. This can lead athletes to crave less-healthy foods and gain weight, apart from reducing energy storage (glycogen) in muscles needed for athletic performance.

Just as sleep improves physical performance in sports, it also improves mental performance—the quick thinking needed for accurate decision-making. This includes skills like interpreting the behavior of opponents, knowing when to change direction and where to aim, and predicting the intentions of your teammates and opponents. Finally, sufficient sleep also improves mood and helps to manage emotional concerns that may interfere during the stress of competition.

Athletic training often requires mastering new motor techniques, which are skills reinforced by one common feature of sleep—sleep spindles, the electrical activity associated with forming and retaining new memories, like motor skills. Sleep spindles are most common during early morning sleep, so setting the alarm too early may reduce the skill learning benefit of sleep. Recent research found that among adults and teenagers learning to juggle, getting sleep after practice led to quicker success, and this learning was associated with sleep spindles. So, if you are a gymnast developing a new floor exercise routine, a good night's sleep after training may just help you land that new flip.

Athletes know that good nutrition, practice, workouts, and stretching are needed for peak performance, but research shows even elite athletes don't get enough quality sleep. Even when sleep is valued and its priority is understood, late-night practice, competition stress, jet lag from competition-related travel, and sleeping in unfamiliar places can all wreak havoc on maintaining a healthy, consistent sleep schedule. Given this, it comes as no surprise that elite athletes often report feeling sleepy during the day.

For peak athletic performance, medical professionals recommend that athletes practice good sleep hygiene above all. That includes sleeping and waking at around the same time each day, creating a comfortable sleep space, and getting seven to nine hours of sleep nightly (or more for teenagers). Although daytime naps can make it harder to fall asleep at night, the rare use of a short nap may temporarily increase alertness to compensate for travel-related sleep disruption if it is completed at least eight hours before bedtime.

Finally, jet lag significantly affects athletic performance, so taking a rest day or more to acclimate to a new time zone is recommended. Prioritize eating and sleeping in the local time immediately on arrival but keep in mind that it takes the brain about one day to adjust one hour—hence, with a three-hour time zone difference it would take about three days to recover from jet lag. Travel from west to east is more challenging because it requires earlier wake times, but getting outdoors in the bright morning sunlight may help reset one's circadian rhythm.

Although even a night of sleep deprivation can challenge athletic performance, all things considered, it is long-term, consistent use of healthy sleep habits that best supports mental, physical, and cognitive health. Healthy sleep habits help to optimize athletic performance over time.

## 14. Does sleeping help you learn and remember things?

Sleep is essential for learning and memory. During the early 1900s, a wannabe millionaire sold a product called a Psycho-Phone, which claimed to enable a person to efficiently learn new information by listening to it play recordings while they were asleep. This product came from the false belief that sleep is like hypnosis, a state of mind when the brain is suggestible and open to new information. However, these theories were debunked during the 1950s by scientists who determined that the only way people could remember information presented to them at night was if they were awake. Furthermore, so-called sleep-learning devices like Psycho-Phone emit sounds that cause brief, unmemorable, but nevertheless harmful awakenings throughout the night, which ultimately disrupts sleep and learning.

Despite marketing promising to help sleepers do everything from learning to speak Spanish to quitting smoking, there is no evidence you can learn information played to you while asleep. But sleep is critical for remembering because it assists with two aspects of learning. First, sleep prepares the brain for learning. Then, in a process called consolidation, sleep allows the brain to move new information from short-term to long-term memory storage, which permits it to be recalled at a later time.

Getting enough good quality sleep prior to learning improves focused attention, making it easier to take in new information. Well-rested individuals can more easily utilize memory techniques and mentally rehearse new information, something called encoding. For example, rather than ineffectively trying to learn the names of 10 people through simple repetition, a well-rested person can more easily come up with ways to recall information by elaborating on the names to be remembered. For example, "Edward: Ed, Ed, his shirt was red, he was pre-med." Someone who is unrested and not fully attentive will not naturally absorb information and will not rehearse information or find useful memory devices. In other words, learning will take longer and will be less accurate.

Research now shows that sleeping after new learning helps move information from the brain's short-term storage to its long-term storage. In turn, people who sleep soon after learning are more likely to recall that information than those who don't. In one recent research study, three groups of people intensively studied new material, with one group napping afterward, one group continuing to study, and one group taking a break. The napping and studying groups remembered the most material, and a week after the study session, those who had napped recalled the material better than the other two groups. The conclusion is less about napping specifically but more generally that the sooner we go to sleep after learning, the better. Studying new material closer to bedtime (but not within the final hour before bedtime, when relaxing is key) improves later recall.

Sleeping for a sufficient length of time is also critical to learning. A recent study found that, compared to those who sleep at least nine hours, school-age children sleeping less than nine hours nightly have more problems with learning associated with physical changes in brain regions responsible for memory and intelligence. Sleep helps us learn and retain new physical skills as well, as discussed in Question 13. For example, when people learned to juggle for the first time, they learned and retained their new skills better if they had the opportunity to sleep after their practice.

During sleep, the brain sorts through the events and thoughts of the day, retaining what is important for long-term memory and letting go of irrelevant information. In the first hour of sleep, heart rate and breathing slow down and people enter what is called Stage N2 sleep. This stage of sleep is marked by a unique brainwave electrical activity called a sleep spindle, which occurs when the part of the brain responsible for new learning (hippocampus) sends information to the outer part of the brain responsible for thinking, problem-solving, and long-term memory storage (cerebral cortex). During rapid eye movement (REM) sleep, when dreaming is most common, brain chemicals help the hippocampus erase unnecessary memories, link memories in new ways, and manage emotional memories. As discussed in Question 10, REM sleep may also support creative thinking and mental health.

Students often ask how best to balance sleep needs against studying demands. People remember the most information when learning new material gradually over time—rather than at the last minute—and when prioritizing sleep consistently to help store new material for the long term. But life is unpredictable and no one has an ideal lifestyle, so sleep needs occasionally conflict with academics. If this occurs, regular breaks for stretching and moving around during late-night study sessions help maintain alertness. While caffeine may also help temporarily, it leads to dehydration that can worsen fatigue, so hydrating with water and limiting caffeine is important.

When sleepiness is difficult to resist during an all-night study session, take the hint and aim to get at least 1.5–2 hours of sleep (i.e., one full sleep cycle) to boost alertness. If only a few hours are available for sleep, going to sleep while it is still dark and waking after sunrise may ease the process of awakening after insufficient sleep. For a morning exam, setting multiple alarms to awaken is likely as necessary as making time for recovery sleep the next night.

## 15. What is the relationship between sleep and mental health?

Good sleep and strong mental health go hand in hand, but the opposite is true as well—mental health problems and poor sleep are closely connected. For a long time, it was assumed that emotional problems were responsible for sleep troubles, but it's understood now that sleep and well-being mutually influence each other—poor sleep hurts mental health, and mental health problems jeopardize sleep, increasing the likelihood of insomnia and other sleep disorders.

As the saying goes, "waking up on the wrong side of the bed" and feeling irritable is common after a single night of bad sleep. Too little sleep also leads to overreaction to negative events—it makes you more likely to lose your temper or misinterpret bad experiences. By making it harder to manage emotions, insufficient sleep increases the likelihood of a person experiencing depression, poor self-esteem, and anxiety. Lower energy levels may also cut into time spent with friends and family, further increasing feelings of being lonely and unsupported.

Common day-to-day worries—such as concerns about school, work, relationships, or money—can interfere with falling and staying asleep. People living in unsafe or uncomfortable situations also have difficulty in letting the body naturally fall asleep. When general life worries are combined with chronic worries about not getting enough sleep, the stage is set for insomnia (i.e., difficulty falling or staying asleep, or waking up too early) to develop.

Those with mental health disorders such as anxiety, depression, bipolar disorder, attention deficit disorder, and post-traumatic stress disorder (PTSD) are very likely to have sleep problems. In one research study, a surprising 95 percent of people aged 7–16 who were hospitalized for mental health problems had abnormal sleep. In another study of adults, 50–80 percent of people treated in a psychiatric practice had chronic sleep issues, compared to fewer than 20 percent of the general population.

There are many ways in which mental health problems could impact your sleep. Often, people who are depressed either sleep excessively or experience insomnia, feeling too sleepy during the day to manage school or work, sleeping at inappropriate times, or waking earlier than desired and remaining awake. People with anxiety may be so focused on worries that they are essentially stuck in a state of long-term stress called hyperarousal—a state of physical and mental activation that overrides the body's natural sleep systems. Those with PTSD also experience lasting states of hyperarousal combined with other disturbances like nightmares or night terrors (episodes of screaming or apparent fear during sleep, see Question 27).

In bipolar disorder, people have periods of either mania (extremes of high energy and overactivity, with little to no desire for sleep) or depression (when they sleep excessively or suffer from insomnia). Interestingly, changes in sleep patterns often precede the symptoms of mania or depression in bipolar disorder. Among people with a history of depression or PTSD who have recovered, the presence of ongoing sleep problems increases the likelihood of these disorders returning in the future. These findings show how mental health problems and sleep problems exist in a vicious cycle in which one reinforces the other.

Rapid eye movement (REM) sleep helps us manage the emotional ups and downs of the past day by sorting through our emotional reactions to events, discarding some memories and sending others to long-term storage. One theory suggests that REM reduces the link between negative events and our intense emotional reactions to them. That is, REM helps us to "forget" some negative emotions from the previous day and to wake up emotionally balanced for the next day having "slept it off."

Although we have our most vivid and emotional dreams in REM, the significance of dreams for managing emotions is not fully understood. Across the sleep cycles in a normal night of sleep, REM periods increase in length toward morning. So, those who don't get enough sleep and awaken early may lose the early morning REM benefits to emotional health. For those with PTSD in particular, nightmares replaying the trauma-related events disrupt REM and result in awakening, making it harder to resolve the negative emotions related to their traumatic experiences.

The close relationship between sleep and mental health offers some positive opportunities for treatment of emotional problems. Treatment that emphasizes getting regular and sufficient sleep helps treat depression, bipolar disorder, and PTSD and reduces the likelihood of these problems returning. For those with PTSD, sleep quality and quantity can be improved by focusing exclusively on the treatment of nightmares using a psychological treatment called imagery rehearsal therapy. In turn, PTSD severity often decreases and sometimes is entirely eliminated through the improvement of sleep alone. Counseling approaches such as cognitive behavioral therapy (CBT) and cognitive behavioral therapy for insomnia

(CBT-I) focus on changing both negative thoughts and sleep habits and have been shown to improve both mental health and sleep.

## 16. How does sleep affect our relationships with others?

Think for a moment about your closest friend and what makes that relationship so special. It may be the sharing of interests and activities or a funny story that only they could understand. It may be that each of you seems to know when the other needs a helping hand and just what to say. It may be that you haven't always gotten along but you've always been able to work out your differences. It probably never occurred to you that your sleep figures in good relationships, but sleep matters a lot in all the above examples.

Now imagine that trustworthy friend cancels your plans at the last minute, and you are feeling disappointed and frustrated. If you are well rested, it is easier to calmly accept the situation by reminding yourself that they rarely flake out and are under a lot of stress. But if you haven't slept much, you probably won't be so forgiving. A lack of sleep makes us impatient and irritable, much like an overtired and moody four-year-old. Sleep loss also makes us less understanding with others, more likely to blame them, and less likely to accept responsibility for our side of problems.

Scientists have found that when we are sleep-deprived, we don't easily see things from others' point of view during personal conflicts. We struggle to read others' facial expressions or accurately understand their state of mind. Our relationships suffer when sleep loss drives us to lose our temper more often, act more impulsively, and be less likely to back down and apologize in an argument. Even a single night of impaired sleep increases conflict in romantic relationships. Couples living together often feel less satisfied with their relationship overall when one has, or both have, inadequate sleep. Sleep-deprived partners may have less interest in intimacy, sex, or family engagement due to lower energy levels. Luckily, after only a night of recovery sleep, the couple is more likely to be harmonious.

As discussed in Question 16, people with sleep problems are more likely to have emotional problems. They may be too tired to socialize, distracted, or simply uninterested in what others are saying. These behaviors may lead others to wonder if the person is harboring a grudge or is bored with the relationship, and they may feel offended about it. When questioned about the cause of their actions, people feeling tired, stressed, anxious, or depressed may not have enough self-knowledge regarding what is going on inside them to explain their feelings, which provides little relief to others. Put another way, it can be hard to be a friend to others when you have ongoing mood or sleep problems, but it is probably a little harder for others to be friends with you.

Loud and frequent snoring is a sign of sleep apnea, a kind of disordered breathing discussed in Question 18. Snoring may be accompanied by sounds of gasping, snorting, and frequent, brief awakenings. Teens who snore sometimes avoid sleepovers or group trips, as the snoring is embarrassing and disturbs others' sleep (see the case study "There's a Big Bear in the Tent"). Some adults in committed relationships even resort to what the popular press calls a "sleep divorce." This occurs when the two people concerned sleep in separate beds or separate rooms because of one partner's sleep problems, remaining in a committed relationship but losing the comfort and intimacy of sleeping together.

Safety is another issue relating to relationships and sleep. Sleep contributes to a significant number of vehicle accidents and puts both driver and passengers at risk. For example, people who sleep less than four hours have a 11.5 times greater risk of getting in a car crash, which helps explain why drowsy driving accidents are more common than accidents caused by drugs and alcohol combined (see Question 37 for more information on drowsy driving). Sleep deprivation also contributes to workplace accidents and can be a particular risk when people have rotating night-shift jobs. It follows that coworkers may be less trusting or comfortable working with people who are drowsy on the job.

Just as bad sleep causes problems for the sufferer, it simultaneously disrupts their relationships. So, take others' sleep needs seriously—just as you wouldn't push a friend to go out in cold weather with just a T-shirt on when they have the flu, you shouldn't push them past their bedtime at night. For those whose sleep apnea–related snoring makes them an outsider, remember that there are very effective treatments. Research shows that after successful treatment of sleep apnea, couples' sleep quality improves, they have fewer disagreements and more "cuddling," and they are happier with their relationships.

## 17. How is sleep influenced by my period?

Many young women who menstruate have trouble with sleep around the time of their period. About a quarter of young women report sleep problems just before the period and a third have sleep troubles during their period. Throughout the first half of the menstrual cycle, hormones build up and support the development of an egg inside a follicle; this is called the follicular phase. At around day 14 or the mid-point of a 28-day cycle, ovulation occurs—that is, the ovaries release a mature egg. This heralds the start of the luteal phase, and if the egg is not fertilized, hormone levels gradually drop, eventually triggering monthly menstruation. Premenstrual symptoms, including sleep issues, are most likely during the late part of the luteal phase, from four to six days prior to menstruation to the first couple of days of menstruation.

About 15–20 percent of young women report a full premenstrual syndrome including mood changes, anxiety, cramping, and bloating. Compared to young women who do not report those premenstrual symptoms, those with premenstrual symptoms are twice as likely to have sleep troubles during the luteal phase. Typical sleep-related symptoms include difficulty getting to sleep, waking up at night, feeling less refreshed in the morning, and daytime sleepiness and fatigue.

Scientists studying sleep across the menstrual cycle believe that shifting levels of the hormone progesterone influence premenstrual sleep changes. When progesterone builds during the luteal phase, it increases normal body temperature by almost 0.7°F. Since late-evening drops in body temperature normally help ease people toward bedtime, this slight increase in body temperature may lead some women to feel uncomfortably warm and have subsequent difficulty getting to sleep. Also, progesterone may cause sleep to shift to a higher proportion of light sleep than normal (NREM Stage N2), leading to less refreshing and restorative sleep.

Hormones influencing the menstrual cycle also affect parts of the brain related to mood, which may account for the stress and mood changes experienced by some women. In addition, especially for girls with heavy periods, worries about staining their sheets or bedclothes, or awakening to change tampons and pads or to empty cups, further disrupt sleep. Finally, menstrual cramps may reduce the depth of sleep and increase awakenings throughout the night.

Although we don't fully understand the cause of disrupted sleep and daytime sleepiness before and during periods, some strategies have been successful in managing these issues. Some women need more sleep during the luteal phase, which is a normal and predictable part of the menstrual cycle. In these instances, this sleep need can be met by increasing time in bed by one or two hours (i.e., by getting to sleep earlier at night, remaining in bed later in the morning, or taking a brief nap in the late-morning hours). Keeping a cooler sleep environment improves sleep quality in general and may counteract period-related increase in body temperature.

Severe menstrual cramps may require further medical tests or medications that can ease the discomfort. But in less severe cases, some sleep benefits have been seen when cramps are managed with a warm bath, yoga stretches, or the use of a hot water bottle or heating pad, or by sleeping in a fetal position. Reducing salt and sugar intake, increasing calcium, and getting more outdoor light may help women experiencing premenstrual symptoms to sleep better.

Finally, research has shown that women who sleep less than six hours a night are more likely to have irregular periods and are much more likely to experience heavy bleeding during their period. So, women should remember that the unwanted sleep-related side effects of their period are temporary and, if they prioritize getting enough good quality sleep, they will soon feel better.

# Sleep Problems, Disorders, and Unusual or Embarrassing Experiences

### 18. What is a sleep disorder, and which sleep disorders are most common in teenagers?

Everyone has problems sleeping occasionally. The most common reason for poor sleep is not giving it high priority and making time for it. According to polls published over several decades, most U.S. teenagers do not get enough sleep. More than 60 percent of young people do not even get the minimum recommended eight hours of sleep on school nights and and insufficient sleep is worse among high school seniors and African American youth.

But despite making time to sleep, some people still cannot achieve a sufficient amount of quality sleep. When this sleep problem continues over a long time, interfering with regular daytime activities and causing frequent sleepiness despite the person having regularly slept for seven or more hours, a sleep disorder may be present. More than 100 sleep disorders have been named and they fall into a few general categories. Some of the most common ones among teens and young adults are insomnia, delayed sleep-wake phase disorder (DSWPD), sleep apnea, restless legs syndrome or periodic limb movement disorder, narcolepsy, nightmares, sleep paralysis, night terror, and sleepwalking.

Insomnia disorder, which is experienced by up to 40 percent of teens, is marked by lasting difficulty getting to sleep, difficulty staying asleep, and/ or waking up too early in the morning. Most people with insomnia report that worry and stress contribute to their problem by overriding the body's natural sleep systems. Over time, daily worries and stress are made worse by worries about not getting enough sleep. The most successful treatment for insomnia is called cognitive behavioral therapy for insomnia (CBT-I), a short-term therapy that combines sleep education, strategies for relax- ation, and set schedules for time in bed. This treatment is discussed in depth in Question 23.

Later bedtimes are typical among teens due to a delayed evening release of the brain chemical melatonin (as explored in Question 9). But this natural pressure to delay bedtime conflicts with school, work, and social obligations that require teens to wake up early in the morning, before they have had a full night of sleep. As a result, about 14 percent of teens strug- gle to wake up on time or to achieve the required number of hours of sleep needed for normal sleep and work activities. If these problems are lasting, interfere with daily activities, and are not better explained by any other sleep disorder, DSWPD may be considered. DSWPD is a type of circadian rhythm sleep disorder, a group of sleep disorders that occur when the body clock becomes mismatched with life obligations.

Obstructive sleep apnea (OSA) involves frequent pauses in breathing during sleep, wherein the pauses temporarily block the flow of air and briefly awaken the sleeper. Sleep apnea is associated with snoring, loud breathing or gasping during sleep, and multiple awakenings throughout the night. Next day fatigue, poor concentration, headaches, and irritability are com- mon (see Question 25 for more on snoring and treatment of OSA). OSA occurs in 1–6 percent of children and adolescents. Breathing temporarily stops during OSA because the muscles and other tissues of the mouth relax and close down the airway. The disorder is more common among children and adolescents with enlarged tonsils, asthma, or allergies that inflame or swell the airway. Across all age groups, being overweight is a major contrib- utor to OSA (30–60 percent of obese teens show signs of OSA).

Nightmares and sleepwalking are two sleep disorders that fall under the category of parasomnias, which are uncommon events or experiences occurring either during sleep or in the transition between sleeping and waking. Most teens have nightmares occasionally, especially during times of high stress or insufficient sleep, during illness or fever, or after taking certain medications. But if the nightmares occur several times a week over a period of time, and if the nightmares are not believed to be the result of a traumatic event or some kind of medication, a formal diagnosis of nightmare disorder is considered. Nightmare disorder occurs in about 7 percent of teens, making it quite common, although its prevalence drops off in adulthood. Like nightmares, sleepwalking is a parasomnia common among children and teens. It occurs in as much as a third of children under 13 years of age but becomes less common toward adulthood. Sleepwalking involves any of a variety of purposeful movement behaviors during deep, slow-wave NREM sleep, with typically no memory of the event the following day. Although sleepwalking is common in teens, hearing about it from others can be very embarrassing. There is no single cause of sleepwalking, but it is more common among family members of people who sleepwalk and is more likely to occur during periods of stress, fever or illness, or sleep loss and after consuming certain medications or alcoholic beverages. Luckily, sleepwalking often resolves on its own over time and requires no formal diagnosis or treatment. Managing sleepwalking, like managing nightmares, requires maintaining regular sleep habits and getting sufficient sleep.

Restless legs syndrome involves unpleasant sensations in the legs (or arms) in the evening and night, accompanied by a feeling of needing to move the limbs to reduce the sensations. Although present in only around 2 percent of children and teens, early identification is important because symptoms can disrupt sleep and often continue into adulthood. Narcolepsy is another rare sleep disorder affecting less than 1 percent of the population. Aspects of sleep and wakefulness overlap in narcolepsy (e.g., severe daytime sleepiness, unintentional napping, temporary loss of muscle control, etc.). Narcolepsy and its related symptoms are often inherited and run in families. Although it begins during the teenage years in half of all cases, narcolepsy is usually not detected until adulthood because it shares symptoms with other more common sleep problems.

### 19. How do doctors measure sleep and diagnose sleep disorders?

When sleep problems continue despite making time for it with good sleep habits, an undiagnosed sleep disorder may be responsible. If a lack of sleep makes it difficult to go to school or work and have a normal social life, it may be time to see a sleep specialist. The first appointment usually involves a thorough clinical interview to explore sleep concerns and patterns, lifestyle, mood, medical history, and overall health. Oftentimes an interview—with questions addressing the main symptoms of sleep disorders—is all that is needed to reach a diagnosis.

The clinical sleep interview might begin with the doctor asking the patient to describe their current sleep problems and having them complete sleep symptom questionnaires. The following are some of the most important questions to be answered:

1) Are you having difficulty getting to sleep, waking up in the middle of the night, feeling excessively sleepy during the day, or waking up too early? (i.e., insomnia, excessive sleepiness)
2) Do you snore heavily or have difficulty breathing at night? (i.e., sleep-related breathing disorders)
3) Are you experiencing bad dreams or night terrors? Do you wake up feeling paralyzed and unable to move? Do you find yourself sleepwalking or having other odd movements or behaviors during sleep? (i.e., parasomnias or sleep-related movement disorders)
4) Do you find it nearly impossible to successfully complete all required activities of work, school, social, and home life due to sleep difficulties?

Particularly if these problems seriously challenge daily functioning, one should take it that with every "yes" in response to the above questions, the greater the likelihood of a possible sleep disorder. If the reader of this book endorsed many of these questions, a doctor's visit is likely in order.

To understand typical sleep patterns, the doctor will ask about the patient's usual bedtime and wake time, daily amounts of sleep, and how much the sleep schedule varies across weekdays and weekends. To assist with this, keeping a sleep diary for a week or two to record sleep and wake times is commonly requested. While there is no universal standard sleep diary, a simple online search can yield many useful options (e.g., the Two-Week Sleep Diary of the American Academy of Sleep Medicine). Some patients are asked to wear a watch-like device called an actigraph for several weeks, particularly when circadian rhythm–type sleep disorders are suspected. This measures movement during one's waking and sleeping hours to estimate sleep duration, and it has recently been integrated into other consumer electronics devices.

A good sleep interview will also look out for major recent stressful events or changes in routine that can alter the ability to sleep, such as concerns about relationships, changes in school or work schedules, illness or death in the family, or mental health difficulties. Other questions explore sleep habits, environmental factors (e.g., bed comfort, noise level, lighting, and sense of safety), and typical routine in the two or three hours prior to bedtime to identify activities that may be delaying sleep (e.g., use of electronic devices, late meals, and vigorous late-night exercise).

The clinical interview also explores the strategies that are already being used to cope with sleep problems (e.g., which bedtime strategy helps you wind down best after a stressful day). People commonly cope with drowsiness using caffeine, taking naps, or trying to make up for lost sleep on weekends. Although these strategies result in a short-term increase in alertness, they also decrease sleepiness at bedtime and can unintentionally make it harder to fall asleep. When coping strategies undermine improvement and progress, they are called "perpetuating factors" since they drive or reinforce the problem. It is critical to identify such perpetuating factors in the interview.

Sometimes, people have unrealistic expectations or inaccurate ideas such as "I can easily catch up on sleep if I miss a few days" or "normal is eight hours of sleep without waking up" (see Common Misconceptions). These beliefs may be tested during the interview as well. Medical history including current medications, assessment of daytime fatigue (energy levels) and sleepiness, physical examination, evaluation of caffeine and recreational substance use, and routine blood tests may also be gathered or considered.

When certain sleep disorders are suspected, an interview alone is not enough for diagnosis but, instead, a formal sleep study is required. These disorders include sleep-disordered breathing disorders (e.g., sleep apnea), narcolepsy (requires both overnight sleep study and in-clinic nap testing the following day), some types of parasomnias like rapid eye movement (REM) behavior disorder, and sleep-related movement disorders (e.g., periodic limb movement disorder and restless legs syndrome). The sleep study, called polysomnography, is usually conducted overnight in a sleep clinic but may be conducted at the patient's home in some instances.

Prior to bedtime, sensors are attached to the body and used to measure breathing, muscle tension, eye movements, heart rate, and sound throughout the sleep period. Changes in each of these sensors help clinicians determine when sleep occurs and how deeply (e.g., the occurrence of frequent eye movements while sleeping is a sign of REM sleep). One of the primary ways of measuring sleep is by using scalp sensors that measure electrical pulses, sometimes called brainwaves. As billions of brain cells communicate during sleep, shifts in their rhythmic, repetitive patterns of electrical activity throughout the brain can be seen, which correspond with different stages of sleep. Following the sleep study, all sensor data is reviewed to determine stages of sleep and the presence of disordered sleep.

Sleep clinicians combine the results of the clinical interview, sleep diaries and questionnaires, physical exams, and laboratory tests to diagnose most sleep problems, although in some instances an additional sleep study is required. Sleep is measured most directly using a sleep study with multiple bodily sensors. Alternatively, sleep can be measured indirectly by estimation using movement (actigraphy) or by using consumer electronic methods of measuring sleep, explored in the next section, Question 20.

## 20. How do watches and other wearable devices that measure sleep work, and should I use one?

Although in-lab sleep studies are the gold standard for measuring sleep, they are also expensive, uncomfortable, inconvenient, and, often, not an option or medically unnecessary. So, affordability, comfort, and convenience drive the wide range of sleep devices seeking to provide an alternative to the formal sleep study. These consumer sleep technologies comprise a wide range of products for people who wish to learn about and improve their sleep, and demand is growing rapidly. The company Graphical Research forecasts that by 2027, sale of sleep devices in North America will bring in annual revenue exceeding $17 billion.

We use "sleep device" to describe this wide category of consumer sleep technologies, which include but are not limited to wearable devices (e.g., watches, rings, headbands, or electronic sleep masks), contactless "nearable" devices (e.g., under-mattress, sheets, or pillow movement sensors, bedside radio-wave frequency motion detection, echolocation tracking), and mobile device "apps." Wearable devices often include actigraphy, which measures movement. Basically, long periods of inactivity are assumed to be sleep, and movement is assumed to reflect wakefulness.

Other sensors are often included to help confirm these assumptions. Both wearable and nearable devices may assess pulse, blood pressure, eye movements, breathing rate, body position, or snoring. This sensor data is combined and analyzed to create user reports which claim to provide information on the length, stages, and depth of sleep, awakenings, activity during sleep, and so forth.

Whether or not to purchase and use a wearable may be best decided by a consideration of the benefits and limitations of these devices. To highlight these, imagine how you might respond to this common scenario: after using a recently purchased sleep tracker for one week, you notice that the device reports very different sleep quality from what you believe occurred. Perhaps it says you are sleeping well despite the fact that you are not feeling refreshed and have been remaining awake for hours at night. Or, on the other hand, perhaps your "good sleeper" identity is shattered by a sleep report showing poor quality sleep. In these instances, you may wonder if the machine is more accurate than your own perception and question whether to make an appointment with a medical provider.

Sleep devices are inherently less precise, accurate, and clinically useful than a professional sleep study. But addressing the specific accuracy of sleep devices is difficult because the answer would vary for each device, software updates and hardware improvements are regularly released, and new products hit the rapidly expanding sleep market annually. Another barrier to answering the accuracy question is that most sleep device manufactures do not disclose precisely how their products estimate sleep to protect secret, financially valuable company information.

Moreover, in an effort to avoid the in-depth oversight process required in the United States to sell "medical devices," manufacturers often avoid government oversight by marketing their sleep devices as "lifestyle/entertainment" devices. Clinicians obviously cannot use entertainment products for medical diagnoses or treatment, and this paired with the lack of manufacturer transparency regarding the formulas used to measure sleep on their devices leads clinicians to often disregard data from sleep devices.

One of the biggest and unexpected drawbacks of sleep devices is that they can create and continue sleep-related problems. Returning to the earlier example of the device reporting sleep data contrary to your perception of your sleep, an inaccurate device may disguise or miss real sleep problems. This would provide inaccurate reassurance and would reinforce the belief that medical follow-up is unnecessary, which ultimately allows the sleep problem to continue. Alternatively, if the device suggests sleep problems are present, regardless of accuracy, this often causes people to worry more about their sleep. Anxiety about sleep, or a purposeful effort to force sleep commonly seen in this situation, often intensifies sleep difficulties.

In fact, the clinical term orthosomnia has recently emerged to describe a condition where people striving for perfect sleep become overly focused on data from sleep devices, which increases anxiety and problems related to falling and staying asleep. This suggests that people prone to worry or with a history of insomnia are risking an increase in anxiety by using sleep devices and so might want to avoid them. If a sleep device is utilized, users are encouraged to avoid checking any backlit screens at night (e.g., a phone app), if applicable, because that can disrupt the natural body clock and delay sleep. Even if no screen is present, checking the device at night is not recommended as this tends to increase wakefulness and anxiety and can cause difficulties returning to sleep.

The recent development of orthosomnia also reflects a common 21st-century myth that "perfect" sleep should occur nearly instantaneously on getting into bed and that it should result in one completely undisturbed eight-hour chunk of sleep. Of course, in reality, healthy and normal sleep takes about 15–20 minutes to start and goes through regular and brief interruptions throughout the night, roughly every 90 minutes. How much a sleep device reinforces the myth of instantaneous and uninterrupted sleep and pushes the consumer toward unrealistic striving for perfect sleep varies by manufacturer but should also be considered before purchase.

Despite these drawbacks, sleep devices have some benefits at both the population and individual levels. From the perspective of broader public health, these devices have helped increase public awareness about the importance of sleep. Sleep devices that provide sleep data in a game-like manner, where digital badges or rewards can be earned by improving sleep, introduce the topic of healthy sleep to a wider audience in a fun and engaging way, raising awareness on the importance of sleep.

Using population data, an extremely large amount of consumer sleep data could theoretically be collected anonymously and analyzed, using computer modeling and artificial intelligence to reveal previously unknown predictors of sleep difficulties before the difficulties occur. While such use of "big data" analysis may lead to insightful and novel community-based efforts to address sleep problems, there are important legal and ethical questions to address regarding control of personal data access, privacy, consent, and so on.

At the individual level, the largest benefit to using a sleep device—besides simply having fun with it—is that it serves as an important reminder to work toward prioritizing sleep. With all the distractions, responsibilities, and entertainment in our modern world, the sleep need is easy to ignore. For better or for worse, sleep devices keep our attention on sleep. This can backfire when unnecessary anxiety is created, as discussed, but the increased attention benefits us when it reminds us to prioritize sleep.

Some devices also provide individualized sleep-timing recommendations based on scientifically supported techniques. Many guide individuals toward making behavioral changes to develop sleep hygiene. Finally, sleep devices may uncover sleep concerns that were previously unknown, leading the consumer to seek out medical assistance that they would not have otherwise sought.

In the near future, as accuracy improves and government clearance is obtained, these devices will likely become more integrated into the medical care system. This could mean long-term data collection to track changes over time, alerting clinicians to unforeseen problems before they arise (i.e., red flags), signaling the need for an appointment, and improved remote communication between patient and provider. This would be particularly useful in places where sleep professionals are underrepresented, like rural areas.

## 21. Why am I sleepy all the time?

People often use the words "sleepy" and "tired" as if they were the same thing and interchangeable, but medically these are different because they have separate causes. Sleepiness, discussed in greater detail in Question 4, is caused primarily by the natural buildup of the chemical molecule adenosine within the brain. This acts like a sleep fuel by obstructing brain cell activity responsible for wakefulness, thereby causing sleepiness. Signs of sleepiness might include a strong drive to go to sleep with difficulty maintaining wakefulness, a feeling of heaviness in the eyelids, yawning, microsleeps or momentary lapses into sleep, or accidental napping such as falling asleep during class.

On the other hand, tiredness is physical, emotional, or mental fatigue. For example, after intense exercise, most people will feel physically tired but not sleepy—in fact, many feel more alert. After taking a challenging final exam, one might feel mentally tired or drained but not likely on the verge of sleep. Signs of tiredness might include perceived low energy or a "dragging" feeling, low motivation, difficulty concentrating, or exhaustion.

There are many potential causes of daytime tiredness, including boredom, medication side effects, not drinking enough water (i.e., dehydration), spending too much time inactive, unhealthy diet, excess physical activity, being overweight, and eye fatigue from spending too much time looking at computer screens. Other potential causes include medical conditions (e.g., low blood pressure, hypothyroidism, low blood iron levels, infections) and mood difficulties (e.g., depression, anxiety, irritability, grief, stress).

When true sleepiness is present during the daytime, two primary brain systems working separately but in parallel are likely to blame: the homeostatic drive and the circadian rhythm. These internal biological mechanisms result from several brain structures and chemicals that drive our wakefulness and need for sleep over time.

The homeostatic drive, or sleep drive, refers to the gradual buildup of adenosine over the course of wakefulness. Due to rising levels of adenosine throughout the day, the longer you are awake, the sleepier you will tend to feel. Once a person is asleep, adenosine is removed from the brain, so you are more likely to awaken feeling refreshed if sleep length is adequately long. But when people do not get enough sleep, which in teens is around nine hours most nights of the week, adenosine is not cleared out of the brain completely. As a result, we awaken feeling sleepy and this sleepiness will be more noticeable throughout the day.

The circadian rhythm is an internal body clock that releases a variety of brain chemicals which suppress sleep and increase wakefulness, as discussed in detail in Question 9. After lunch, particularly between 1:00 p.m. and 4:00 p.m., the alerting signal from the circadian rhythm is reduced temporarily until it increases again in the early evening. As a result, we all experience a midafternoon dip in energy during which the sleep drive (adenosine) becomes more noticeable while the wake drive (circadian rhythm) is less powerful. It may come as no surprise that napping cultures around the world, particularly in warmer climates, time their naps or siestas around this natural post-lunch dip in alertness and increase in sleepiness.

Hot afternoon temperatures can cause feelings of sluggishness or tiredness as the body uses up significant energy trying to cool itself. Sweating can sometimes lead to dehydration and lower blood pressure, which intensify fatigue. So, struggling to stay awake after lunch results from a combination of this physical fatigue and the increased sleepiness and related drop in body temperature from the natural midafternoon dip in the body's circadian rhythm. For more information on the circadian rhythm, see Questions 9, 22, 24, and 42.

In addition to lack of sleep, another cause of daytime sleepiness is having a sleep disorder that causes poor quality sleep, interfering with adenosine removal during sleep. Sleep disorders often disrupt the normal cycles and depth of sleep and cause awakenings. Sleep-related breathing disorders like sleep apnea and sleep-related movement disorders like periodic limb movement disorder are conditions associated with daytime sleepiness, as discussed in Questions 23, 25, and 26.

Narcolepsy is another sleep disorder associated with daytime sleepiness, although excessive adenosine is only half the story. Orexin is a small chemical protein that promotes wakefulness throughout the brain, but people with narcolepsy lack brain cells that produce this protein. Due to a lack of orexin to offset the drowsiness-inducing effects of adenosine, people with narcolepsy feel constantly sleepy and often accidentally but rapidly fall asleep throughout the day.

## 22. Why do I have so much trouble getting to sleep at night?

There is rarely a single root cause to difficulties falling asleep. Instead, a wide variety of factors cause these problems, which can intensify over time. To help make sense of the many factors influencing sleep issues, doctors use a "four-factor model of insomnia." The four factors include predisposing factors, precipitating factors, perpetuating factors, and conditioned arousal. For many people, focusing on the first three factors is enough to improve sleep. However, if problems falling asleep continue over weeks or months, it becomes necessary to address conditioned arousal, the final factor.

When exploring the possible sources of the problem, the first consideration is looking for any biological or psychological characteristics that place a person at higher risk for sleep difficulties. These are what doctors call "predisposing factors," and they may include things like demographic factors, genetic or medical conditions, and personality characteristics. Demographic factors include differences in sex, ethnicity, and age—for example, adolescents experience a natural delay in the body clock that results in a biological preference to delay bedtime whereas older age is associated more with unpleasant leg sensations that delay sleep (restless leg syndrome). Difficulties falling asleep can be inherited, as can many other sleep disorders, so considering family history is also important. Lastly, people who tend to be anxious are more likely to think about daytime worries—and about the problems they are having with their sleep itself—at bedtime, both of which increase alertness and delay sleep.

The circumstances that led to, or relate to, the first appearance of sleep difficulties are referred to as the "precipitating factor." Other precipitating factors include recent increases in life stressors (e.g., job or academic stress, relationship problems, changes in health) or emotional turmoil (e.g., anxiety, depression, grief over the death of a loved one). People with mental health difficulties are more likely to have trouble falling asleep, so the onset of mental health problems may be a triggering factor.

Changes in one's habits, such as increasing caffeine consumption, altering timing of meals, or decreasing physical activity, may lead to difficulties in falling asleep. Medical or physical changes such as long-term pain conditions or diabetes can also trigger similar problems. Recreational, alcohol and nicotine, and prescribed medications that disrupt sleep (e.g., steroids, appetite suppressants, antidepressants) may also need to be adjusted, changed, or eliminated with the guidance of a doctor. Finally, environmental factors like bright light exposure at night, disruptive noise, inappropriate sleeping temperature, safety concerns, and unsuitable setting can all delay sleep if not addressed.

Changes in sleep timing, due to beginning a night-shift work schedule, for instance, or due to jet lag following air travel across time zones, is a common precipitating factor causing difficulties in falling asleep. As discussed in Question 9, the circadian rhythm is our internal clock that regulates sleep timing. When this system is disrupted, sleep gets disrupted. Common pitfalls include exposure to bright or blue light after sundown (e.g., TV and computer screens), failure to keep a consistent bedtime and wake time, and inadequate overall daytime light exposure.

Once difficulties falling (or staying) asleep become frequent, people may turn to certain habits or behaviors that they believe will help them cope but that actually make the problem worse. Examples are sleeping in on the weekends to "catch up" on sleep, napping more frequently, trying to force sleep (e.g., counting sheep), drinking caffeine excessively to manage daytime sleepiness, drinking alcohol near bedtime as a "nightcap" sleep aid, and so on. However, these "perpetuating factors" often make the sleep problem worse over time and are the third factor to consider when addressing difficulties falling asleep. Recommendations for how to develop healthy habits and behaviors for sleep, which address most of these perpetuating factors, are discussed in Question 40.

Some people who have problems falling asleep report that getting into bed brings on uncomfortable emotions, regardless of how relaxed they felt just before that. Many of these people feel anxious or nervous after getting in bed while others report fear, anger, worry, frustration, and hopelessness. Whatever the negative emotion may be, these feelings are highly alerting and delay sleep. Similarly, thoughts may be calm prior to bedtime but, once in bed, become active and stressful (e.g., "Not again! How long will it take me to fall asleep tonight? If I don't, tomorrow will be ruined.")

This experience is explained by the fourth factor known as "conditioned arousal." This final, and exclusively psychological, factor occurs when the bed and bedroom are no longer associated with sleep. Ideally, our brain thinks of the bed as a place for sleep, sex, and relaxation. But in conditioned arousal, after weeks of being in bed awake and frustrated, the brain eventually learns that the bed is a place of stress and wakefulness. As a result, people who develop conditioned arousal may struggle to remain awake while relaxing on the couch before bedtime but suddenly feel wide awake after getting into bed. Thoughts in bed dreading another night of poor sleep also increase wakefulness and agitation at bedtime, further delaying sleep.

Conditioned arousal can be thought of as a self-perpetuating cycle of stress and wakefulness. This cycle can be broken and the problem resolved using a treatment called cognitive behavioral therapy for insomnia (CBT-I), which will be explored further in the next question. Additionally, directly addressing anxiety and stress-related factors is equally important, utilizing techniques discussed further in Question 39.

## 23. Why do I keep waking up throughout the night, and how do I stop this?

Before worrying too much about waking up at night, understand that it is entirely normal for everyone to awaken naturally and periodically throughout the night. In fact, almost everyone awakens briefly about every 90 minutes between sleep cycles, all night long—so roughly awakening five to six times every night. Scientists suspect that changing positions helps prevent blood from pooling in one area of the body, but regular nighttime awakenings may also be a throwback to our evolutionary past—a chance to check for predators near the sleeping environment to determine if it is safe to continue sleeping. Most people return to sleep so quickly following these brief awakenings that they do not even recall it the next day. If something occurs during this natural awakening that activates the brain, however, it increases alertness and creates a memory of the awakening.

For example, checking the time at night involves doing math—how much time has it been and how much time is remaining—which is alerting to the brain. In addition, checking time on one's phone increases the chances of seeing updates or missed messages from others that one believes must be addressed. While the phone itself is largely associated with activities that stimulate the mind, its screens interfere with normal circadian processes, as unhealthy light exposure fools the brain into inaccurately concluding that the sun is rising.

Avoid checking the time at night and consider placing the clock out of reach to decrease the temptation to check it. One may even use reassuring self-talk to shut down unhelpful thoughts during middle-of-the-night awakenings, such as "It doesn't matter what time it is—the alarm clock I set will wake me up. I just need to relax." When seeking clinical treatment for difficulties maintaining sleep, clinicians will likely further explore challenging thoughts about sleep and address misunderstandings, myths, unrealistic expectations, and dysfunctional thoughts.

But when nighttime awakenings reoccur frequently, lasting 30 minutes or more each time, other factors may be causing them. Sometimes, other disorders are responsible for nighttime awakenings. For example, depression is associated with early morning awakenings with difficulty returning to sleep. Sleep disorders like obstructive sleep apnea and nightmare disorder can cause unwanted and frequent awakenings. Finally, many medical conditions and medications are known to disrupt sleep. Speaking with a medical professional is important to sort out these issues.

Other than the reasons just reviewed, one of the most common causes of difficulties staying asleep is conditioned arousal. As discussed in detail in Question 22, conditioned arousal occurs when the bed is associated with stress and wakefulness. When awakening naturally at night between sleep cycles, people with conditioned arousal may check the time, begin to predict poor sleep, and worry about how they will function the next day. These emotions, thoughts, and behaviors in turn lead to worsening sleep.

Conditioned arousal results in difficulties falling asleep and problems staying asleep, but both can be successfully resolved by working with a sleep clinician using a treatment called cognitive behavioral therapy for insomnia (CBT-I). Since 2016, the American College of Physicians has recommended that "all adult patients receive CBT-I as the initial treatment" for long-term difficulties falling and remaining asleep. Their research review led to the conclusion that, compared to sleep medication, CBT-I is as effective in the short term and more effective in the long term, with fewer side effects.

CBT-I combines elements of education, sleep hygiene, stress management, and cognitive therapy to address unhelpful thoughts. Many people misunderstand sleep and have misperceptions that intensify the problem. So, education about sleep-wake systems and normal sleep is critical to eliminate unhelpful beliefs or myths and set realistic expectations at the beginning of CBT-I. This education also focuses on developing healthy sleep hygiene habits by recommending specific lifestyle and behavior changes that promote good sleep (discussed in greater detail in Question 40).

Falling asleep is an involuntary process—it must come naturally and cannot be directly controlled. If people could simply try harder and force themselves to sleep, insomnia wouldn't exist. But when awakened in the middle of the night, some people still try very hard to force sleep by counting sheep, trying to sleep despite not feeling sleepy, drinking a very special tea before bed that "guarantees" better sleep, and so on. When our efforts to force sleep fail, it is frustrating and this makes us more alert. Whether at the beginning or middle of the night, the conclusion is clear: the more we try to force sleep, the less likely we are to achieve it.

CBT-I redirects this effort to controlling that which we can control—our behaviors, habits, and routines, and the timing of our sleep. One of the hardest but most important of controllable actions is getting out of bed at a consistent time. A set of guidelines in CBT-I called stimulus control aims to eliminate conditioned arousal by decreasing efforts to force sleep and by associating the bed with sleep. This occurs by first encouraging people to remain out of bed until they feel sleepy and ready for sleep, or for sex (i.e., ensuring they are not in bed for watching TV, using the Internet, or having conversations about potentially disturbing emotional issues). Once in bed, if sleep does not occur within roughly 15 minutes, people should get out of bed and do something relaxing until they feel sleepy and ready to return to bed.

For middle-of-the-night awakenings, CBT-I recommends remaining in bed at first, if relaxed, but getting out of bed and doing something relaxing if sleep doesn't return shortly—avoid checking the time but take approximately 15 minutes before getting out of bed. Although often frustrating, the reason for getting out of bed is to avoid continuing to associate being in bed with wakefulness. Nighttime activities out of bed should be relaxing or minimally stimulating, and in low light. By limiting the time that one is awake and frustrated in bed, the brain begins to learn and rediscover that the bed is a place for sleep.

The longer someone remains awake, the sleepier they become and the more likely they will be to sleep. Although we cannot force sleep, we can force wakefulness and, in so doing, indirectly influence sleep. This approach within CBT-I was historically called "sleep restriction," but a more accurate description of this technique would be "time-in-bed restriction" since excessive time awake in bed is directly targeted and restricted, not sleep. This sleep efficiency training technique aims to improve sleep quality by increasing the percentage of time in bed spent sleeping.

Based on the amount of actual sleep achieved on a recent average night, clinicians assign a prescribed bedtime and rise time, which usually results in reducing the amount of time spent in bed overall. Although this practice may lead to sleepiness initially, over time the body learns to associate the bed with sleep, overcoming conditioned arousal by limiting the amount of time spent awake in bed. Once good sleep efficiency emerges (defined as sleeping for at least 85 percent of the time spent in bed), the time in bed can be increased by 15 minutes every 5 days until the desired sleep quantity is met. Those interested in trying CBT-I are encouraged to seek out a sleep clinician who can work collaboratively to develop an individualized treatment plan.

As explored in depth in Question 15, sleep and mood influence each other significantly, with difficulties in one area undermining progress in the other. Therefore, in addition to utilizing the stress management techniques discussed in Question 39, people with mood disorders and sleep problems improve most when treating both problems simultaneously.

## 24. What is the best way to fight jet lag and shift-work problems?

You're going from Chicago to Paris for what is expected to be the vacation of a lifetime. After a long overnight flight, you arrive at your hotel at 7:00 a.m., excited to see the Eiffel Tower. But unfortunately, it's midnight in Chicago and your body is all ready to sleep! Despite some coffee and your best efforts to not sleep through most of the 9:00 a.m. bus tour, it happens. Jet lag—a short-term disruption in the daily rhythm of sleep and wakefulness that results from travel across time zones—is to blame.

Symptoms of jet lag include daytime sleepiness, low energy, and a feeling of alertness or sleepiness consistent with the departure time zone but incompatible with the local time. Our body clock influences not only sleep timing but also daily cycles of digestion, body temperature, alertness, strength, mood, and cell growth. So, in addition to sleep difficulties, jet lag often results in feeling unwell, being grumpy, having an upset stomach, feeling overly cold or warm, and other problems.

People vary somewhat but, on average, it takes about one day per time zone for the body to recover its normal rhythms. This tends to be worse during travel from west to east, which requires going to bed earlier on arrival and waking up earlier in the morning. Because the body clock is naturally and slightly longer than 24 hours, it resets each morning with sunlight. This creates a natural preference to delay sleep and wake times rather than advance them (as eastward travel usually requires). Unfortunately, returning home will restart and extend the jet lag symptoms.

To a limited degree, caffeine drinks and the excitement of travel can silence or overpower jet lag. But the best way to overcome jet lag is by using the body's natural timekeeper—sunlight. An hour's walk in the bright morning sunlight (and indoor lights) helps the brain's timekeeper, the suprachiasmatic nucleus (SCN), reset daily to local time. Morning light triggers the SCN to suppress and delay release of the chemical melatonin, helping energize us to jumpstart the day. As daylight fades toward the end of the day, melatonin is released from the brain's pineal gland, making us sleepy and gently easing us toward bedtime.

Knowing this, jet lag is best managed when morning and early-afternoon light exposure is maximized for several days following arrival and evening light (including artificial light from electronics) is avoided at least one hour before bedtime. Also, since people commonly awaken in the middle of the night during jet lag, try to keep the lights dim and avoid use of electronic devices with screens because both delay adjustment to the new time zone.

Strategies employed by veteran travelers include updating watches and clocks on arrival in a new time zone, drinking plenty of water, eating meals and socializing in sync with local time, and avoiding too much caffeine and alcohol, as both of these substances are dehydrating and can make jet lag worse. If possible, a rest day or two is valuable to adjust to the arrival destination before vigorous work, particularly for highly intense physical or mental activities. Finally, some people speak with their doctor about the short-term use of over-the-counter melatonin pills. When timed properly, such as a low dose of melatonin five hours prior to the desired bedtime, this can decrease the time required to adjust to a new time zone.

Now, imagine a college student attending full-time school during the day and also working a job on the "graveyard shift" (midnight to 8:00 a.m.) two or three nights a week, in addition to socializing in between. As the SCN struggles to determine time of day and adjust sleep-wake systems accordingly, the frequent changes in the timing of sleep and wakefulness that result from shift work create a state similar to being stuck in a jet-lagged condition, unable to adjust to a set time. Regardless of possible sleep loss, the quality of the sleep is also likely to suffer with shift work, causing a cascade of health complications over time.

Shift work provides our society with essential services that, for some people, need to be available at night. Unfortunately, this need is also associated with the risks of shift work (i.e., excessive sleepiness, poor mood, relationship problems, and higher risk of obesity and cancer). Other than ending the job commitment or taking time off to let the body recover, management of shift-work symptoms largely echoes the techniques used for jet lag. To minimize the related life and health problems, scientists primarily recommend keeping the same bedtime across the week, even on days off, with an extended sleep period just before beginning a night shift or following a night shift.

Of course, the solutions are unique for each person, considering their usual activity needs over the rest of the day and the rest of the week. Naps, melatonin supplements, and caffeine can help, or make things worse if used improperly, so sleep professionals may be necessary for timing and dose recommendations. When daytime sleep is required, dark or orange-tinged sunglasses and blackout curtains can be used at home to minimize light exposure, and earplugs can block out environmental noise. Finally, some people experiment with interventions to increase alertness during a night shift, like taking a brief nap (i.e., 20 minutes or less), having caffein-ated beverages (i.e., no more than two servings daily, ideally not within 8 hours of desired sleep), or using commercial light boxes (i.e., 10,000 lux at arm's length for 30 minutes) just before a night shift to suppress the brain's release of melatonin.

## 25. Why do people snore or stop breathing in their sleep, is it dangerous, and how can it be prevented?

Snoring is the noisy and rough sound heard when the air we breathe causes vibration of tissues in the throat. Occasional snoring is common, not particularly dangerous (although potentially a sign of danger), and not usually a cause for concern, although it may disrupt the sleep of those who can hear it. Frequent snoring—three or more times per week—occurs in around 15 percent of children and teens and 25 percent of adults. It is associated with greater sleepiness during the day and can lead to concen-tration and behavior problems as well as poorer grades in school. How-ever, when nightly snoring is accompanied by other breathing problems like pauses in breathing, or when it seriously disrupts sleep, it may be a symptom of obstructive sleep apnea (OSA). OSA is the most common sleep-related breathing disorder, occurring in 2–4 percent of the general population.

Snoring is caused by anything that narrows the nasal passages or throat airways and interferes with the flow of air during sleep. On falling asleep, the airway in the throat naturally relaxes, causing it to be slightly reduced in size. In frequently snoring adults, excessive fatty tissue in the airway is often responsible, caused from being overweight. The most common reason for snoring in young people is congestion and inflammation due to a cold, asthma, or allergies. Better management of these conditions may likely reduce or eliminate snoring.

Problems in nose and throat structures may also be responsible, like enlarged tonsils and adenoids or elongated soft palate (the rear roof of the mouth) or uvula (the tissue that hangs from the back of the mouth). Snoring can also be caused by a deviated septum, which occurs when the tissues between the nasal passages are pushed off to one side, blocking one of the nasal passages. Finally, anything that relaxes the muscles in the tongue or throat during sleep can partly block the airway and cause snoring. This may be an inborn condition like genetic airway size or a temporary result of not getting enough sleep.

Rather than being directly treated and eliminated, snoring is primarily managed and prevented. Snoring is typically worse when one sleeps on the back, so "positional therapy" aims to avoid this by taking steps to either sleep on one's side or elevate the upper body with various pillows (because breathing is generally easier when one is upright). Pillows between the knees and behind the back may be used to encourage side sleeping; on the other hand, sleeping with a small backpack with a tennis ball inside could discourage sleeping on the back. Alcohol is a depressant that should be avoided before bedtime because it relaxes the muscles of the mouth and throat extremely effectively, increasing snoring and breathing difficulties while ruining sleep quality.

If other conditions are responsible for snoring, a doctor may prescribe allergy or asthma medications or decongestants to ease nighttime breathing. Less effective solutions include nasal strips on the bridge of the nose to slightly widen the nostrils and ease breathing or exercises to strengthen the muscles of the mouth and throat (e.g., opera voice lessons). Often, doctors recommend avoiding nicotine, increasing exercise, and weight loss to reduce excessive tissue in the airway. Alternatively, surgery might be recommended to remove excessive tissue or if the structure of the jaw, mouth, or nose is responsible for OSA.

While snoring isn't inherently dangerous, it can signal the presence of the dangerous underlying disorder called OSA, particularly when accompanied by pauses in breathing while asleep, called apneas. When breathing stops and oxygen drops, it signals the brain to wake up and breathe. These apneas trigger brief awakenings accompanied by gasping or snorting sounds as breathing resumes. People with OSA may have hundreds of these apneas on any one given night, often with no memory of it the following day because the awakenings are too short to form a memory of them. Given this lack of awareness, OSA symptoms are typically first reported when witnessed by the bed partner or family members.

Arguably, it would be a form of torture to awaken somebody briefly but repeatedly, every 12 minutes or less, anytime they try to sleep. But OSA literally does that. This lighter, less restful sleep stresses the heart and interferes with normal and necessary sleep-related health maintenance, and its effects carry over to daytime (i.e., sore throat, morning headache, severe sleepiness, difficulty concentrating). Over time, untreated OSA can lead to higher risk for a number of dangerous diseases, including high blood pressure and heart problems.

Doctors evaluating for severe snoring or signs of OSA typically examine the nose and throat visually to check for factors that narrow the airways, like infections, enlarged glands, and signs of allergy. Sometimes a doctor will request an X-ray scan or other tests to look for any problems in the structure of the jaw, throat, and nose that could be causing the symptoms. They may also recommend wearing a simple device called an oximeter for a period of time, which can measure the level of oxygen in the blood while a person is sleeping to determine effectiveness of breathing. Finally, as described in Question 19, a formal sleep study may be ordered to monitor breathing and sleep stages throughout the night.

Prevention of OSA mirrors what was previously introduced for snoring. But treatment for sleep apnea varies depending on its cause. If obesity is believed to be the primary contributor, an exercise and weight loss program will likely be advised (somewhat unfairly, as OSA commonly results in further weight gain, as discussed in Question 12). When airway obstruction causes apneas, a continuous positive airway pressure (CPAP) machine is usually prescribed because it is the most effective treatment available. This is a special breathing device that delivers lightly pressurized room air through a mask, which keeps the airway open and reduces apneas.

If apneas are caused by the central nervous system occasionally skipping breaths (i.e., central sleep apnea), oxygen therapy or variable pressure level therapy (i.e., BiPAP) may be considered. Although people sometimes find the CPAP machine awkward at first, adjustments to the mask and device settings can help with comfort and fitting it to an individual. When sleep apnea is in the mild range, and particularly when CPAP has been difficult to tolerate, a variety of oral appliance devices that open the airways during sleep are offered by some dental providers in lieu of CPAP.

To summarize, snoring may be a nuisance but is not generally a concern unless it is frequent and severe or if it is accompanied by signs of OSA. The best strategy is to avoid alcohol a few hours before bedtime and to avoid sleeping on the back. Although sleep apnea can have serious long-term health consequences, it can be effectively treated by working with a medical provider. For a description of a teen with OSA, see the case study, "There's a Big Bear in the Tent."

## 26. Why do some people kick or move around in their sleep?

Ask someone on the street what healthy sleep looks like and a common response would likely be: A healthy sleeper falls asleep nearly instantly after getting in bed, then remains asleep and essentially motionless for roughly eight hours, awakening only once in the morning feeling refreshed. But this notion is flat-out wrong. In reality, healthy sleepers fall asleep after about 15–20 minutes; in fact, falling asleep in under five minutes is a sign of possible sleep disorders or not getting enough sleep. Healthy sleepers also awaken naturally about every 90 minutes, for brief periods throughout the night. One purpose of these regular awakenings is to adjust body position to avoid muscle soreness and ensure essential blood flow to all parts of the body.

So even the healthiest sleepers naturally move, periodically, throughout sleep and the movements may sometimes be kicking movements. Another kick-like movement can occur when we are falling asleep. People sometimes report sudden, involuntary muscle contractions or twitches in the limbs or body when falling asleep, and these are known as hypnic jerks or sleep starts. Sometimes, they are described as feeling the need to catch oneself from falling out of bed and may be associated with hallucinations (seeing or hearing things that are not there). Hypnic jerks are not a medical concern but are often a sign that the person is not getting enough sleep.

Another common cause of movement is muscle twitches during dream sleep, as the urge to act out dreams sometimes breaks through the mechanism working to prevent us from hurting ourselves. Finally, young children may rock themselves to sleep or have rhythmic movements of the body or head, moving side to side or rolling. While rhythmic movements in bed are common among young children, they normally stop naturally by age five and are generally not a cause for concern. However, a sleep-related rhythmic movement disorder may be diagnosed if this behavior continues past age five and results in injury, poor sleep quality, or difficulties like sleepiness the following day.

In some instances, however, sleep-related movements are caused by a sleep disorder. At bedtime, people with restless legs syndrome (also known as Willis-Ekbom disease) have difficulties falling asleep due to uncomfortable feelings in the legs described as "creepy-crawly," "a deep itch," "tingling" or "electric" sensations. While leg movement provides relief from these sensations, the urge to move also delays sleep. Once asleep, about 80 percent of these individuals also have periodic limb movements or periodic limb movement disorder (PLMD), which may further disrupt sleep quality.

Sleep-related movement disorders like PLMD are simple, repetitive, involuntary movements that disrupt sleep quality. Periodic limb movements typically last between one-half of a second and ten seconds and can occur sporadically or in a repetitive pattern. When these occur more than 15 times an hour in adults or more than 5 times an hour in children, a diagnosis of PLMD may be considered.

Teeth grinding or clenching while asleep, also known as bruxism, is another movement disorder explored in Question 33. Although scientists do not yet fully understand the nature of the relationship, bruxism is known to be extremely common among people who also have a sleep-related breathing disorder. People struggling to breath while sleeping often move during these moments, gasping for air with a twitch, kick, or adjustment in sleeping position. So proper treatment of underlying sleep disorders like obstructive sleep apnea can indirectly end both bruxism and frequent nighttime movements.

All the above instances refer to involuntary movements that are brief and simple, like a twitch. When movements during sleep last greater than 10 seconds and behaviors appear more complex or organized, parasomnia-type sleep disorders may be responsible. Such behaviors like sleepwalking and sleep talking are further reviewed in Question 31.

## 27.  What is the difference between a nightmare and a night terror?

While nightmares can be terrifying, a night terror is clinically distinct from a nightmare and has nothing to do with dreaming. The clinical definition of a nightmare is repeated awakening from sleep with a detailed recall of extremely frightening or threatening dreams. These dreams are associated with an intense fear, awakening and placing the body on high alert for rapid response to potential dangers (i.e., the "fight-or-flight response"), which delays the person's return to sleep. Nightmare dream content may be rapidly forgotten, interfering with later recall, but it still causes significant distress or impairment. Nightmares are most common in the second half of the sleep period when rapid eye movement (REM) sleep is most likely. On the other hand, night terrors, also known as sleep terrors, occur when the sleeper appears awake and extremely fearful (e.g., eyes open, flailing arms, talking or yelling out) but remains technically asleep. Unlike nightmares, these episodes are not associated with dreaming in REM sleep and occur earlier, usually several hours after initial sleep onset. If awakened by others during the event, people become confused and disoriented; however, the individual is unlikely to recall the event the next day if left undisturbed. Notably, night terrors are fairly common in children and not usually a sign of mental health problems.

Among adolescents and younger adults, women report more nightmares than men, and during childhood, girls experience more night terrors. When nightmares are repetitive and reoccurring, some individuals will begin to delay going to bed to avoid experiencing nightmares. However, this results in sleep deprivation, which is a major risk factor for nightmares and night terrors. In fact, because nightmares disrupt sleep quality and night terrors can result from sleep disruption, nightmare occurrence is itself a risk factor for and increases the risk of developing night terrors.

Night terrors are classified as parasomnias, which are experiences (e.g., hallucinations, strong emotions) or undesirable events (e.g., sleepwalking, sleep eating) that occur while asleep or during the transition between sleep and wakefulness. Other types of parasomnias are sometimes mistaken for night terrors or nightmares. When transitioning between different stages of sleep, some people awaken feeling an immediate sensation of danger and threat that appears similar to the "fight-or-flight response" seen following nightmares. These nocturnal panic attacks are distinct from nightmares in part because there is no recognizable dream content recalled and, unlike what happens with night terrors, the individual is awake during the event.

Historically, the word "nightmare" was not used in reference to a disturbing dream but rather described a parasomnia we today call sleep paralysis. The early 14th-century word "mare" described an evil female spirit who lay on and suffocated sleepers (of note, this "night mare" does not relate to the modern definition of a mare, a female horse). Sleep paralysis episodes are commonly described as awakening and having awareness of one's surroundings and wakefulness, while simultaneously feeling extreme terror, sensing an "evil" presence, and feeling a terrifying crushing or pressing sensation on the chest with trouble breathing and difficulty moving. In other words, when transitioning from REM sleep to awakening, some individuals become temporarily stuck between stages and essentially display characteristics of both wakefulness and dream sleep. See Question 28 for more information on sleep paralysis.

## 28. Sometimes at night I see or hear scary things in my bedroom, and I cannot move at all—am I going crazy?

Probably not. Hallucinations occur when people report seeing, hearing, or otherwise perceiving things that others cannot confirm or perceive. Although hallucinations can be a sign of mental illness, they are also quite common—particularly in bed—and not necessarily cause for major concern. Dreaming is a type of hallucination. While not everyone can recall their dreams, scientists have discovered that everyone dreams while in rapid eye movement (REM) sleep. That is, everyone hallucinates on a nightly basis.

Other hallucinations that are associated with sleep and not necessarily cause for concern are hypnagogic hallucinations, which occur while falling asleep, and hypnopompic hallucinations, which occur during the process of waking up. These fleeting hallucinations include sensations that are not real, like sounds, sights, or the physical experience of touch, and are fairly common among teenagers and adults. Less commonly, sleep paralysis may occur simultaneously with these hallucinations during the transition into or out of sleep. During sleep paralysis, people are fully aware of their sleeping environment and wakefulness, but at the same time, they are unable to move their body or speak. This is often associated with feelings of intense fear and, similar to hypnagogic and hypnopompic hallucinations, seeing visions or hearing things that are not actually present in reality.

Sleep paralysis reflects an overlap between wakefulness and REM sleep, as if the sleeper is temporarily stuck between the two stages. REM sleep is distinguished from wakefulness by several key features, including rapid eye movements, dreaming, increased activation in the brain's emotional center (amygdala), and the loss of normal skeletal muscle tone. This temporary paralysis of voluntary controlled muscle groups typically prevents people from acting out dreams and becoming hurt or awakened. Therefore, all the key features of sleep paralysis (i.e., immobility, hallucinations/dreams, high emotionality) arise out of normal changes associated with REM sleep, albeit while awake and oriented to one's surroundings.

Throughout history, the signs and symptoms of sleep paralysis were explained through the cultural lens of its time and place, often by referencing evil spirits, witchcraft, or supernatural creatures. For example, people from the United Kingdom and Newfoundland have historically described a witch or "old hag" who sits on the body of a sleeper, which in the southern United States has come to be called being "hag ridden." Other tales and creatures of the night used to explain sleep paralysis include rapist demons known as incubus and succubus, a *"kokma"* attack where dead children supposedly attempt to choke sleepers (St. Lucia, West Indies), or the sleeper being "ghost covered," what is called *"phi um"* in Thailand.

A modern example of using a cultural framework to understand sleep paralysis can arguably be seen in the typical alien abduction story: awakening and sensing the presence of a nearby alien or threatening entity, being strapped down to an alien operating table or feeling unable to move and frozen in place by alien technology and extreme fear. The sexual undertones often included in alien abduction stories, like being impregnated or probed, similarly echo the sexual aspects seen in many cultural explanations previously.

Sleep paralysis cannot be directly treated, and hypnagogic and hypnopompic hallucinations are a relatively harmless and normal occurrence that do not require treatment. So, clinicians focus instead on eliminating or reducing triggers to sleep paralysis, which include times of high emotional stress, times when one is sleeping less than seven hours most nights, times when one has a fever, and times when sleep quality is disrupted, for instance due to medications, alcohol, drugs, or untreated sleep disorders like sleep apnea.

## 29. Why do I have "wet dreams" or wake up in the morning with an erection?

People often falsely assume that an erection on awakening is a result of sexual dreams or desire or, alternatively, a strong urge to urinate. Dreams are most likely to occur in rapid eye movement (REM) sleep and this stage occurs more frequently and for longer durations toward the end of the night. Regardless of dream content or subject, genital blood flow naturally increases during REM sleep. This results in morning awakenings with a REM sleep–related erection, sometimes called "morning wood," and is entirely normal. In fact, this is a sign of good heart and genital health. Notably, women experience similar genital blood flow changes during REM sleep but these are less visible.

Among adults, about 8 percent of dreams contain sexual content. So, unless specific sexual imagery is recalled, an erection on awakening is rarely a result of dreams. Approximately 4 percent of dreams result in orgasm, according to one study. When men orgasm during sleep and ejaculate, doctors call it a nocturnal emission; among the general public, this is known as a "wet dream." A similar experience in women may cause vaginal wetness and awakening.

A wet dream may occur at any time after the onset of puberty, but it is most common among teenagers and young adults. Some men experience this after abstaining from masturbation or sex for one to two weeks, although the frequency of these episodes varies greatly depending on the person. About 40 percent of women and 80–90 percent of men report experiencing at least one wet dream. People with more frequent wet dreams tend to be those who are sexually inactive, particularly those who masturbate less often or abstain altogether.

In conclusion, while sexual dreams may cause an orgasm or an erection on awakening, these are most often caused by entirely normal and healthy REM-related physical changes. Realistically, there isn't a way—or a need—to stop waking up with erections. While wet dreams cannot be fully controlled, some people find that increasing masturbation frequency can help avoid nighttime orgasm; however, cultural or religious guidance may prohibit this.

## 30. Sometimes I pee in my bed while asleep—how can I stop doing this?

Bedwetting, called nocturnal enuresis by clinicians, occurs when a person involuntary urinates while sleeping. This is common in young children who are still learning bladder control and being toilet-trained, but bedwetting typically stops naturally over time. For example, only about 10 percent of 7-year-old children experience bedwetting and this percentage continues to fall; by age 15, only 1–2 percent experience bedwetting.

A family history is a very common risk factor for bedwetting; for example, you would have a 70 percent chance of developing bedwetting problems if both your parents had this same difficulty. In these instances, family members are encouraged to be patient and understand that the sleeper is not to blame for something they did not intend to do. Shaming or punishing bedwetters leads to self-doubt and stress, which usually makes the problem worse over time. However, struggling with bedwetting can in itself be very stressful, embarrassing, and harmful to self-esteem for some individuals. In such cases, people often benefit from speaking with a counselor or therapist to address concerns.

When bedwetting occurs after childhood, emotional or psychological functioning is often normal, although there is a greater presence of recent life stressors (e.g., moved to a new school, family relationship issues).

While the connection is not totally understood, people struggling with bedwetting are more likely to also have attention deficit hyperactivity disorder. Medical issues like diabetes or urinary tract infection are considered as possible causes but are rarely to blame. People with a sleep-related breathing disorder like obstructive sleep apnea are at a higher risk of bedwetting, so effective treatment of the underlying sleep disorder may resolve bedwetting. Sleepwalking has also been linked with nighttime urination when the sleeper falsely believes they are near a toilet.

Behavioral management strategies include avoiding consumption of a lot of fluids in the evenings and using the toilet immediately before getting into bed. People struggling with bedwetting are encouraged to avoid all liquids two hours prior to bedtime. They need to avoid caffeine and alcohol in particular because these increase the urge to urinate. Although not a solution, use of waterproof mattress pads or diapers marketed as "absorbent underwear" or "incontinence briefs" for adults can help manage cleanup the following day.

When seeking professional assistance, physicians may offer medications that reduce bedwetting, such as tricyclic antidepressants, or in more extreme cases, surgery (i.e., urethral dilatation). Desmopressin is another medication that works very effectively by limiting the production of urine during sleep. Some clinicians may recommend scheduling awakenings periodically throughout the night, such as by recommending an alarm to awaken the sleeper every two or three hours to urinate.

While doctors and patients have found scheduled awakenings to be useful, this is not strongly supported in the research. What is strongly supported is the use of a bedwetting alarm and pad system, which can be purchased over-the-counter. These devices are placed under the person in bed and will sound an alarm to awaken the sleeper once any moisture is detected. At first, this results in awakening following a few drips of urine rather than after full emptying of the bladder. But over time, this trains the brain to recognize the sensation of a full bladder and eventually learn to awaken naturally to use the bathroom.

## 31. Why do people sleepwalk or talk in their sleep, and is this unsafe?

Sleepwalking and sleep talking are the most common of all parasomnias and are generally safe. Parasomnias are abnormal actions or behaviors that occur while a person is asleep or in the transition between sleep and wakefulness. Some parasomnias are relatively harmless and common, while others can be unpleasant or dangerous to the sufferer and their bed partner. Some parasomnias only occur in rapid eye movement (REM) sleep, such as REM behavior disorder and nightmare disorder. Non-REM (NREM) parasomnias include sleep terrors, confusional arousals, and sleepwalking, among others. Given this, scientists know that sleepwalkers are not acting out their dreams because the behavior does not occur in dream sleep (i.e., REM).

Although the brain is technically in deep sleep while sleepwalking (stage N3), individuals appear awake to outsiders and move around the environment with eyes open. All NREM parasomnias, like sleepwalking, occur most commonly in the first third of a night's sleep. If awakened during the event, people will often be confused, fearful, disoriented, or sometimes violent. However, if left undisturbed or softly encouraged to return to bed, sleepwalkers will have no memory of the experience the following day.

Traditionally called somnambulism, sleepwalking occurs in 29 percent of children aged 2–13 years with most events occurring between ages 10 and 13. About 4 percent of adults report ongoing sleepwalking. In contrast, sleep talking is very normal and occurs occasionally in most individuals. Other parasomnias like sleep talking are variations of the same mechanisms leading to sleepwalking. These involuntary sleep behaviors may include sleep eating (i.e., sleep-related eating disorder), sleep sex (i.e., sexsomnia or sleep-related abnormal sexual behavior), sleep driving, and so on.

During a confusional arousal, people may speak in a confused or incoherent way that sounds like sleep talking. In these instances, people awaken from NREM sleep feeling confused; they remain in bed, speaking slowly or minimally, and are less responsive to the environment. In adults, this lasts for 5–15 minutes, but children may sit up in bed for up to 30 minutes whimpering or moaning. In either case, people are generally inconsolable but should nevertheless be spoken to quietly, reassured of their safety, and gently encouraged to return to sleep.

The most common triggers for sleepwalking are not getting enough sleep regularly, recent stressful life events, or recent strong positive emotions. So, sleepwalking can be avoided by improving stress management, sleeping at least seven hours every night, and keeping a consistent sleep-wake schedule. Other recommendations, though less effective, are avoiding intense exercise before bedtime and reducing alcohol, caffeine, and use of recreational drugs.

Sleepwalking may be triggered by some medical conditions (e.g., fevers in children, migraine headaches, stroke) or sleep medications known to increase the risk of parasomnias (especially sleep-related eating). Sleep disorders that disrupt normal sleep stages can also trigger sleepwalking, in particular, sleep-related breathing disorders like sleep apnea. Finally, sleepwalking can be genetically passed on and occurs more often during the premenstrual period, following travel across time zones, and when sleeping in unfamiliar, noisy, or bright surroundings.

For the most part, sleepwalking is harmless and serious injury only occurs in very rare circumstances. Although asleep, there is a small level of brain processing reserved for safely navigating the real-world environment while sleepwalking. However, in some cases, sleepwalkers have injured themselves or others. This can result from, for example, falling downstairs or into the pool, walking through a glass door, mishandling dangerous or sharp objects, operating machinery or vehicles, or walking onto an active roadway. Rather than treating the underlying problem, many people focus on making the environment safer to avoid injuries. These changes could include sleeping alone, locking doors or windows, moving breakable items or tripping hazards, wearing restraints, placing weapons or car keys out of reach or locked away, and, for children, avoiding the top bunk and considering use of a stairway gate.

Other parasomnias carry similar safety concerns, such as sexually transmitted disease or unwanted pregnancy following sleep sex as well as poisoning or weight gain following sleep eating. These conditions can create serious relationship stressors and possible risk to one's bed partner. For example, sleep talking may be disruptive to partner sleep quality and the sleeper may also say things they would not share if awake, leading to embarrassment, anger, or relationship stress. In rare instances, people have carried out complex, dangerous, and illegal behaviors while asleep—including murder. Question 32 explores the topic of violent sleep behaviors, and the legal complications it creates, in greater detail.

## 32. Is it true that people can do violent things in their sleep?

In 1987, following a period of significant life stress, Canadian Kenneth Parks drove 20 kilometers, assaulted his father-in-law, and killed his mother-in-law. Although he drove to the police station later that night and confessed to the crimes, Mr. Parks was ultimately acquitted and not held responsible for his actions because he was sleepwalking. A sleep study showed irregular brain activity consistent with his claims and the good relationship he had long maintained with his in-laws offered no alternative motive. The "sleepwalking defense" has been accepted in U.S. law since the Albert Jackson Tirrell case of 1846, in which a man was found not guilty for arson and killing his mistress while sleepwalking. Although controversial, sleepwalking is an uncommon defense and has been used with variable success.

As discussed in Question 31, sleepwalking is a type of non–rapid eye movement (NREM) parasomnia that can be associated with violent sleep behaviors. However, violence is most commonly seen among people with rapid eye movement (REM) behavior disorder, 64 percent of whom have assaulted or injured their bed partner. REM sleep is normally associated with a loss of muscle tone called paralysis, which prevents dreamers from moving and acting out dreams. But in REM behavior disorder, people physically and vocally act out dreams due to a lack of normal REM muscle paralysis, which can sometimes result in physical injury or violence to self or others.

Applying sleep science to criminal acts, such as in the investigation of violent and strange behaviors during sleep, is known as forensic sleep medicine. Experts in forensic sleep medicine assess patients and may conduct laboratory sleep studies, provide consultation to legal professionals, and offer expert testimony in courts. Although a common concern is that criminals may abuse this defense and "fake it," it is rarely seen in courts because parasomnias cannot be faked when their presence is being verified using a clinical sleep study.

If someone has no desire or intention to harm others but involuntarily does so while asleep and unconscious, some experts would argue they are not responsible for these actions. On the other hand, skeptics argue that people do have some control over their actions while asleep, such as putting on clothes or engaging in conversations while sleep talking. Unquestionably, people have a responsibility for their daytime behaviors, and certain daytime choices may increase risks for parasomnias, for example, keeping an inconsistent sleep schedule, not setting aside enough time for sleep, using alcohol or drugs, not addressing mental health problems like stress, and so on. In these instances, one could argue there is some degree of personal responsibility for parasomnias and their consequences. So, the use of the sleepwalking defense has been, and remains, controversial.

While it is true that some people do violent or illegal things while asleep, it is luckily very rare. When it rises to the level of legal intervention, violent or dangerous behaviors have been attributed to REM sleep behavior disorder, sleepwalking, insomnia disorder, narcolepsy, confusional arousals, sleep sex, nightmare disorder, sleep terrors, and sleep driving. These sleep disorder defenses have had mixed success in court, with the majority of cases relating to accusations of sexual assault, followed by intoxicated driving, homicide, and assault.

### 33. Why do I grind my teeth while sleeping, and how can I stop it from hurting my jaw in the morning?

Teeth grinding and jaw clenching while asleep is called sleep bruxism. Many are unaware of the cause of their morning soreness but learn of these sleep behaviors from others who heard the scraping, clicking, grinding, crunching, or popping noises at night. Sometimes, dentists notice worn down tooth surfaces or even tooth fractures during a routine appointment; these are suggestive of bruxism, particularly if patients report jaw pain or morning headaches. Bruxism can occur as early as infancy and last until older adulthood, but it is quite common in young people. Researchers disagree about how common it is among children, with estimates varying from 10 percent to 49 percent.

Bruxism is not in itself a dangerous condition and may cause no significant harm if it occurs only occasionally. However, if it recurs over time, it can wear down tooth enamel, causing broken and misaligned teeth or sensitivity and pain when consuming very hot or cold food or liquids. Of greatest concern is when it causes jaw pain, earache, or headache due to the tension caused by frequent clenching and the muscle tension in the jaw, which can also disrupt sleep and daytime functioning. It can also contribute to a condition called temporomandibular joint disease, in which pressure on the jaw joint makes it swollen or painful. Finally, bruxism is also a nuisance and a potential sleep disruptor for others who have to witness the sounds of teeth grinding.

Doctors believe that stress and anxiety—especially academic and work concerns—can trigger jaw clenching and teeth grinding during sleep. However, higher levels of daily stress among people with bruxism are not always confirmed in research, so other factors likely contribute. Bruxism is more common among boys, among those with misaligned teeth, among children who have been exposed to secondhand smoke, and among those who tend to breathe through their mouths rather than their noses. Obstructive sleep apnea (OSA) is one sleep disorder associated with bruxism; however, it is unknown whether OSA is the cause or a consequence of bruxism. Nevertheless, treatment of OSA often reduces or eliminates bruxism symptoms.

When bruxism is mild and only occasional, it usually resolves on its own and may need no treatment. However, if dental damage is considerable or if the bruxism causes significant pain and sleep disruption, several effective treatments exist. Nightguards are a variety of simple devices made of thin plastic or acrylic that are molded to cover the surface of the teeth and worn during sleep, thereby shielding the teeth from damage from grinding. While next day jaw pain may still continue with nightguards, the teeth will no longer be damaged. Sometimes, dental treatment is required to repair injury to the teeth.

After a long and demanding day, people may bring their worries and stress to bedtime in the form of muscle tension. Although complete stress avoidance is impossible, stress management is helpful for sleep generally and bruxism specifically. This might include cutting back on extracurricular activities or work or speaking to a counselor about one's stressors and worries. Regular physical exercise, relaxation techniques like diaphragmatic breathing, and meditation exercises can reduce one's overall stress, as can adopting a comforting bedtime ritual each night such as writing in a journal, taking a warm bath, or listening to soothing music. Gentle massage of the facial muscles as well as use of warm or cold compresses on the jaw can reduce both jaw pain and sleep bruxism. But if OSA is present, direct treatment of OSA may reduce bruxism, which has been discussed in Question 25.

# Improving Your Sleep

### 34. Which sleep aids are the safest and most effective?

Recent decades have seen a trend toward increased use of all kinds of sleep aids, including prescription and over-the-counter (OTC) medications, natural supplements, and recreational substances. There is an astonishing variety of sleep medications, and a recent survey showed that 8.4 percent of adults in the United States use sleep medications either most days or every day. Although some specialized medications target specific sleep disorders, like nightmares or restless legs syndrome, most sleep aids target symptoms of insomnia—aiming to increase drowsiness and support falling asleep. Unfortunately, no perfect sleep aid exists, so each sleep aid is a trade-off between benefits and side effects and risks.

In the United States, prescription sleep aids are medications with standardized dosing that have been approved by the Food and Drug Administration (FDA), which evaluates research on effectiveness and safety. All sleep medications have side effects and risks which vary in intensity depending on an individual's age and health status. Sleep medications are dangerous if mixed with alcohol, recreational drugs, and certain other medications, so they should only be used with a doctor's prescription and guidance.

Depending on their chemical composition, sleep aids work through a variety of mechanisms in the brain. Medications like the "z drugs" and benzodiazepines stimulate the brain chemical GABA to induce sleepiness. Melatonin receptor agonists are synthetic versions of the natural substance melatonin that promotes sleepiness in the brain at bedtime. A newer strategy called orexin receptor antagonists induces sleep by reducing levels of orexin, a brain chemical that supports wakefulness. Medications used for other purposes, such as to treat depression, are also sometimes prescribed to enhance sleep.

Most sleep medications are designed for short-term use over several days to weeks and only occasionally, despite often being used regularly for months to years. When used long term, abruptly stopping some sleep medications can produce unpleasant or dangerous withdrawal symptoms that further disrupt sleep. Many sleep aids also cause a "hangover effect," as chemicals remain in the body into the next day, creating daytime sleepiness and concentration difficulties. Some sleep medications reduce breathing while asleep, which can contribute to risky sleep-related breathing disorders. Older adults in particular are at increased risk for sleep-aid side effects like falls or confusion due to age-related changes in how the body processes medications.

The aisles of pharmacies are filled with an overwhelming selection of OTC sleep aids that can be purchased without a doctor's prescription. Many contain antihistamines originally designed to control allergies, such as diphenhydramine or doxylamine. These medicines are commonly used because they are sedating, cheap, and readily available. However, they are not recommended for extended use because people require more and more of the medicine over time to achieve the same effects (an effect known as tolerance). Unwanted sleepiness from antihistamines also often carries over into the next day.

Herbal and other plant-derived supplements for sleep include valerian, lavender, and cannabidiol, which come in the form of pills, chewable "gummies," powders, teas, oils, and tinctures. Some of these products are based on substances present naturally in the body that have been found to contribute to sleep, like melatonin. Though often marketed and perceived as more "natural" and, therefore, safer with milder side effects and fewer risks, these supplements are not necessarily safe. Unlike medications regulated or approved by the FDA, there is often a lack of scientific evidence regarding the benefits and risks of herbal and supplement products, and dosage may vary across batches or over time since there is no quality control of the kind seen with FDA-regulated medications. Cannabis-based herbal approaches to sleep management are explored in Question 35.

Melatonin is a common OTC sleep aid that mimics the chemical melatonin normally produced in the brain. Although melatonin is thought of as a substance that induces sleep, its work is better described as gently shifting the body clock to support sleep. As noted in Question 9, melatonin regulates the daily timing of sleep and wakefulness. Building up in the brain as sunlight subsides, melatonin helps turn off alerting systems in the brain, easing us gently toward sleep. Melatonin pills work in similar ways, helping people with jet lag or odd shift-work hours in falling asleep, apart from their occasional use by others who need help in falling asleep. However, melatonin supplements are not effective for people with severe insomnia and can cause stomach upsets, headaches, and sleepiness during the day at higher doses.

The safest substances sometimes used to ease into sleep are also the least supported in the research literature. The lavender flower is the source of certain essential oils and some teas containing it claim it helps initiate sleep. Valerian is a herb that has been used since the time of the Roman empire to treat insomnia and anxiety (possibly by extending the sedating effect of GABA in the brain). Two natural substances called tryptophan and 5-HTP may also support sleep by increasing the level of the chemical serotonin in the brain, but there is enormous need for more research.

Finally, occasional alcohol use helps people get to sleep and so it is frequently used as a "nightcap" sleep aid. But alcohol causes lighter and less refreshing sleep. When used regularly and over a long period of time, tolerance develops to the sleep-inducing effects of alcohol, with the person requiring higher amounts to achieve the desired effect on sleep; this can result in psychological or physical dependence on alcohol.

To summarize, short-term and occasional use of sleep aids can help some people fall and stay asleep more easily. Potential side effects and risks include daytime sleepiness, trouble concentrating, or becoming dependent on the medicine to sleep, as some people rely excessively on sleep aids rather than trying to improve sleep in other ways. Both prescribed medications and OTC sleep aids should be avoided in people with certain medical conditions. Given the highly personalized considerations necessary when it comes to medication use and choice, it is important to review treatment options and risks with a doctor.

To be clear, the safest and most effective way to sleep is through maintaining healthy sleep habits and keeping consistent sleep timings, as discussed in detail in Question 40. For people with severe problems falling and staying asleep, lifelong use of sleep medication is not often required. Instead, there are established and effective treatments like cognitive behavioral therapy for insomnia, discussed in Question 23, which can eventually eliminate the need for medication.

## 35. How do alcohol and cannabis affect sleep?

Alcohol is the most commonly used sleep aid worldwide, with even a single serving having the potential to cause feelings of sleepiness. A drink before bedtime often helps people fall asleep more rapidly, but unfortunately, sleep across the entire night will ultimately be lighter, less refreshing, and more interrupted. Poor sleep quality following alcohol use increases risks of mood and stress-related difficulties the next day, which may be coped with by using alcohol in the evenings (thus restarting the cycle). More simply, alcohol is a trickster because it is briefly helpful for falling asleep, seemingly benefiting us, but it ultimately robs us of the quality, deep sleep so critical for health.

Feelings of overall relaxation arise when production of the brain chemical GABA is reduced by alcohol, which is also why alcohol is often used to "de-stress and unwind." Due to its effect on other brain chemicals, as alcohol is digested and processed in the body during sleep, its effect shifts from causing sleepy feelings to increasing wakefulness and light sleep. As a result, alcohol negatively changes the normal depth and timing of the stages of sleep. This explains the common perception the morning after alcohol-influenced sleep: "I think I slept well but I don't feel very rested."

In general, the risk of sleep problems ranges from around 9 percent after fewer than two drinks to 24 percent after two drinks and 39 percent after more than two drinks. In addition, because alcohol tends to be dehydrating, people often need to wake up at least once to urinate or hydrate. Finally, after people drink heavily, they may feel hungover and fatigued the following morning, which is largely due to the sleep disruption and dehydration.

Sleep disruption caused by alcohol results in the same risks and problems seen in any sleep disruption—health problems or difficulty concentrating in school or work. Overuse of caffeine to manage these problems may lead to an unhealthy cycle of caffeine during the day to stay alert and alcoholic beverages at night to relax. Long-term heavy alcohol use can lead to developing tolerance to the sleep-inducing effects of alcohol, with the person requiring higher amounts of alcohol to get to sleep. Sleep disruption including insomnia may become worse, however, after ending chronic heavy alcohol abuse and sleep cycles may take a long time to return to normal, if ever.

To minimize the risk of poor sleep after use of alcohol, people are advised to drink only lightly in the evening and to stop drinking several hours prior to bedtime. As noted in the discussion of snoring and sleep apnea in Question 25, alcohol relaxes the muscles of the throat, mouth, and nose, which can lead to snoring. So those with sleep apnea are at higher risk and are advised to drink lightly or not at all.

More than half of young adults who regularly use cannabis report using it for sleep. Research suggests that cannabis can improve overall quality of sleep, reduce the time taken to fall asleep, and reduce middle-of-the-night wakings in individuals with chronic pain or anxiety. Cannabis can be smoked, vaporized (vaping), eaten, or absorbed using liquids called tinctures, all of which may be tailored to higher or lower doses, and each method will differently affect how much and how quickly it influences sleep. How sleep is influenced by cannabis is not fully understood, but one theory suggests it increases adenosine, the brain chemical that causes us to feel sleepy toward the end of the day.

The cannabis plant contains a complex variety of chemicals that impact the brain and influence sleep, primarily CBD (cannabidiol) and THC (tetrahydrocannabinol). Although THC may cause feelings of sleepiness or sedation at high doses, it likely disrupts the normal cycles of sleep, especially among new users. Like alcohol, THC appears helpful to the user but interferes with normal sleep, such as by reducing time in rapid eye movement (REM) sleep. Compared to THC, CBD acts differently on sleep, with low-dose CBD increasing alertness and only higher doses promoting sleep.

CBD has been found to decrease symptoms of excessive daytime sleepiness, and it may treat some disorders of REM sleep. Other research has suggested that THC may be helpful to reduce the symptoms of obstructive sleep apnea or the severity of nightmares after trauma. When combined, THC and CBD may improve management of medical conditions that harm sleep, such as chronic pain. Different cannabis strains have different terpene profiles, which are compounds that are responsible for the different smells across plants (e.g., pine, citrus, floral). Scientists suspect these terpenes may explain the variety of different effects experienced across cannabis strains, which would suggest that terpenes are responsible for feelings of sleepiness more commonly experienced in certain strains (e.g., Grandaddy Purple, Indica).

But there are many unanswered questions about the use of cannabis for sleep, such as what strain is ideal for sleep, how much should be taken, what is the safest method of ingestion, and whether long-term use ultimately helps or harms sleep. Some research suggests that frequent and long-term users of cannabis have more severe sleep problems than those who use it only occasionally or not at all. Other negative effects experienced by some people include dizziness, anxiety, confusion, and fatigue.

Research into the effect of cannabis on sleep has been limited in the United States historically, but changes in cultural attitudes and the recent shifts in the legal status of cannabis will increase access to it by researchers looking for answers.

When used only occasionally, cannabis or alcohol may help people fall asleep more quickly. But long-term use of any sleep aid, including alcohol and cannabis, is not recommended. This is due to risks of its effects becoming less noticeable over time (tolerance), the potential for needing it—or coming to believe one needs it—to sleep (psychological or physical dependence), less restful and refreshing sleep overall when using it, and increasing difficulties sleeping when trying to stop sleep-aid use. It's important to note that at the time of publication of this book, by U.S. federal law, it is illegal for anyone under the age of 21 to consume, smoke, purchase, or possess cannabis. In addition, cannabis may particularly harm the growing brain of children and teenagers, so they should avoid it.

## 36. How do coffee and energy drinks keep you awake, and can they negatively affect your sleep?

Worldwide, caffeine is the most frequently used psychoactive drug. People have used caffeine products like coffee and tea for centuries to decrease feelings of sleepiness and increase mental and physical energy. As discussed in Question 4, caffeine works by blocking brain receptors for the substance adenosine, a brain chemical that builds up during one's waking hours and contributes to feeling drowsier over time. Caffeine does not eliminate adenosine or reduce sleep need but, like putting on a blindfold, it temporarily blocks the brain from being aware of continually increasing adenosine levels.

When consumed in coffee and energy drinks, it takes only 20 or 30 minutes for us to notice the effect of caffeine. But how much and for how long the caffeine affects us is highly individualized. Some people feel alert and energized, while others feel more jittery and anxious, have digestive problems, or feel like their heart is pounding. Long-time caffeine users develop a tolerance and will require more coffee to get the same effect of wakefulness. Doctors' recommendations vary, but typically, they say that daily caffeine should be limited to between 200 mg and 400 mg. How quickly the caffeine clears from the body also varies. Based on genetics, some people take around 4–6 hours to reduce the amount of caffeine in the body by half, while others can take as much as 8–10 hours. Other factors like medications, tobacco use, pregnancy, and diet may also change how quickly caffeine is cleared from the body.

Energy drinks are beverages claiming to improve alertness as well as mental and physical performance. About one-third of teens use energy drinks regularly, and there are even more users among young adults. Many of those who consume energy drinks are unaware of their many ingredients and their effects. Although energy drinks typically contain a variety of ingredients such as ginseng, guarana, various vitamins and minerals, taurine, and (often a considerable amount of) sugar, caffeine is usually the main ingredient. Energy drinks can contain between 70 mg and 400 mg of caffeine—400 mg is as much as three to four cups of brewed coffee. In addition, some ingredients like guarana contain extra caffeine, and ingredients such as ginseng may also have a stimulating effect. Given the combination of caffeine with additional stimulants, it is not surprising that people feel more alert, and have improved physical endurance and faster reaction times after an energy drink.

Although the body's caffeine response during sleep is different across people, the effect of caffeine on sleep is stronger when it is consumed closer to bedtime. Recent research showed that 400 mg of caffeine consumed even six hours prior to sleep resulted in lighter sleep overall, reductions in NREM sleep, and an average of one hour less sleep over the course of the night. This means that although some people proudly proclaim their ability to fall asleep soon after consuming caffeine, the caffeine is nevertheless hurting their sleep quality (even if they are not aware of it).

Usually, the beneficial alerting effects of coffee and energy drinks last between six and eight hours. When early morning beverages with high levels of caffeine and sugar are digested, the initial boost may turn into a midafternoon energy crash. When afternoon coffee and energy drinks are used to cope with this dip or "caffeine crash," it is likely to take longer to fall asleep, with lighter and less refreshing sleep. In turn, this poor sleep is often managed using caffeine the following day—restarting this unhelpful cycle.

Beyond knowing your body and how it responds, the general recommendation for any type of caffeine consumption is to moderate and limit it. An easy rule of thumb for sleep is to avoid caffeine after lunch (or within eight hours of bedtime) to reduce risk of sleep difficulties. If you have difficulty sleeping at night and you are too tired to make it through the day, beware that the body can become dependent on caffeine after heavy daily use.

## 37. Is a "coffee nap" a good strategy to reduce the risks of drowsy driving?

Vehicle accidents are the leading cause of death among teenagers, and no doubt this is partly due to drowsy driving. A National Highway Traffic Safety Administration survey found that 4 percent of people admitted to falling asleep at least once while driving over the 30 days prior, with one-third of people reporting this had occurred at least once in their lives. The risk of falling asleep while driving is particularly high among male teens and young adults, those who have irregular work hours, and those who have had less than six hours of sleep. Drowsy driving accounts for an estimated one in ten motor vehicle accidents, and teens and young adults are believed to account for half of these.

Most teens are very aware of the risks of drinking alcohol and driving, which is often heavily emphasized during drivers' training. But surprisingly, the evidence shows that drowsy driving accidents are more common than those from drugs and alcohol combined. It turns out that the impact of drowsy driving and drunk driving are quite similar—after around 18–19 hours of wakefulness, driving performance deteriorates to a level comparable to that of someone who is drunk driving (i.e., blood alcohol concentration greater than 0.08).

When drowsy, people pay less attention to the road and are more likely to cross roadway lines. If they must swerve or brake suddenly to avoid an accident, their reaction time is slower and they may not respond in time. Shockingly, drowsy drivers are also prone to "microsleeps," where the brain takes extremely brief naps to make up for lost sleep. Lasting only seconds and often outside the awareness of the driver, the consequence of these brief naps can be lethal because the napper is effectively driving blind. All in all, drowsy driving makes people less able to make good decisions during both routine driving and in sudden, hazardous situations.

As discussed in Questions 36, the caffeine in coffee masks the chemical buildup of adenosine in the brain responsible for feelings of sleepiness, but it does not eliminate adenosine. The only way to reduce feelings of sleepiness caused by adenosine is by sleeping, and even a brief nap of 20 minutes can help. So, the idea behind the coffee nap (aka nappuccino, caf nap, power nap, tactical napping) is to maximize alertness by combining caffeine with sleep.

Ideally, the coffee nap would start with consuming one or two servings of a caffeinated beverage, followed by a nap of no longer than 20 minutes using an alarm. This works best if done in the early afternoon and at least six to eight hours before bedtime to avoid disrupting nighttime sleep. The idea of drinking coffee prior to a nap may not make intuitive sense, but given the typical 20- to 30-minute delay in experiencing the effects of caffeine after consuming it, this allows for the perfect length of nap prior to the caffeine taking effect.

A brief nap is ideal because it eliminates some sleepiness by reducing adenosine, whereas a longer nap can cause one to enter deeper sleep and wake up feeling groggy or disoriented. Some research suggests that sleep from the nap may also boost the effectiveness of caffeine by making the brain receptors for caffeine more available. There are only a few studies on the coffee nap, with significant limitations within the research. However, these studies suggest that the coffee nap measurably increases skills, including performance on a driving simulator, on computer tasks, and on nighttime work. In addition, a coffee nap works better than either coffee or a nap alone, and it also works better than washing one's face after napping, cold air exposure, or bright light exposure.

Returning to the original question directly: Is a "coffee nap" a good strategy to reduce the risks of drowsy driving? The research suggests it might be, but much more research in real-life performance tasks like driving is needed. In addition, although the coffee nap seems to boost alertness and energy, drinking or eating anything during driving leads to the dangers of distracted driving, so it's better to drink coffee before driving. The ideal amount of caffeine, the best time of day, the best length of nap, and the expected time frame of beneficial effects is not known but likely varies considerably between people. What is known is that the safest strategy of all is to avoid drowsy driving entirely, if possible.

Apart from the coffee nap, napping in general can give a needed boost to people in the middle of long work shifts. In 1994, the National Aeronautics and Space Administration (NASA) conducted research on pilots on long-haul and transoceanic flights. They found that pilots performed better throughout the flight, and in particular during the important descent and landing phases, when allowed to take naps in the air, giving rise to the term "The NASA Nap." However, a nap can reduce the buildup of adenosine during the day that increases the pressure to fall asleep at bedtime, causing problems falling and staying asleep.

The afternoon nap is a tradition in many cultures, in particular in warmer climates where people feel a strong dip in energy and alertness in the early afternoon. Following lunch, our circadian rhythm decreases alertness for a period of time called the midafternoon dip. This dip in energy, combined with the buildup of sleepiness-inducing adenosine by midafternoon, naturally lends itself to napping. This tradition is called the "siesta" in many countries, the name originating from the Spanish phrase "sexta hora" or sixth hour. That is, the nap after lunchtime falls about six hours after waking. Some Japanese companies provide employee napping facilities, where napping on the job is considered a sign of a hard worker who is loyal to the company.

In summary, drowsy driving is extremely dangerous and should be avoided. Napping too may have unintended consequences by reducing the pressure to sleep the following night, so naps should be used rarely. The need for daily naps may also suggest that an underlying sleep disorder has not been addressed. When safety is of concern, such as when driving drowsy, short naps and caffeine may have a moderate benefit. But ideally, don't drive drowsy.

### 38. How do my daily habits, like exercise and what I eat, influence my sleep or dreaming?

Greek philosopher Aristotle wrote in 300 BCE that sleep was the result of food digestion. He believed ingesting the evening meal caused "hot vapors" to rise toward the brain and cool down, causing us to fall asleep. According to the theory, when food is fully digested and converted to blood, the new blood heats up and travels to the brain, allowing us to awaken refreshed. Aristotle's theory has long since become obsolete, but it shows how suspicions about the role of diet in sleep have a remarkably long history.

After having gorged on a large feast, people inevitably feel tired afterward. Articles addressing the common post–Thanksgiving meal energy crash often point to tryptophan in the turkey as the source. The brain alters the substance tryptophan into melatonin and serotonin, two brain chemicals that influence sleep. But it turns out that other typical foods (e.g., squash) have even more tryptophan—turkey doesn't really contain much. For example, two 8-ounce glasses of tart cherry juice is a much better source of tryptophan that increases total sleep time. But realistically, it's unlikely that any single meal would offer enough tryptophan to have any measurable effect on sleep. More likely our post-meal fatigue is the result of our bodies working to digest an extremely large meal with high levels of carbohydrates as well as the relaxing effects of alcohol consumed with the meal.

Certain foods consumed near bedtime can disrupt sleep. A spicy meal with a lot of hot pepper can increase body temperature, which disrupts normal temperature drops that help us get to sleep. In addition, among those with sleep apnea, both spicy and acidic foods (e.g., citrus fruits, tomatoes) can cause backing up of stomach acid into the esophagus (acid reflux), which can irritate the throat and worsen apnea symptoms.

High-fat foods (e.g., fried foods, pizza) and high-protein foods like meat take a long time to digest, and when these are consumed just before bedtime, their digestion can increase acid reflux and disrupt sleep. Some people believe fermented and aged foods that contain tyramine (e.g., soy sauce, cheeses, processed meats) may act as stimulants and should also be limited before bedtime. Complex carbohydrates like rich desserts or highly sweetened beverages may increase middle-of-the-night awakenings and reduce depth of sleep. But, a simple carbohydrate snack of oatmeal or a piece of toast is unlikely to interfere with sleep and may be just the thing to ease us into it.

As discussed in depth in Question 13, exercise and sleep are bidirectionally related—sleep can improve the quality of exercise and athletic performance and exercise improves sleep quality. Regular moderate exercise—typically defined as a brisk walk for 20 minutes, five times a week—can improve overall sleep quality by increasing sleep depth, decreasing the time it takes to fall asleep, and reducing the severity of sleep problems like insomnia, sleep apnea, and restless legs syndrome. Exercising consistently at regular times provides a strong cue to the body clock for timing of wakefulness and sleep. The body works to repair tissues and recover from exercise using growth hormone released during slow-wave sleep, increasing pressure for deeper sleep following physical activity.

Sleep recommendations traditionally advised against exercising several hours before bedtime due to it increasing core body temperature, mental stimulation, and, potentially, chemical stimulation (i.e., an "adrenalin rush"). But despite this concern, some researchers have not found sleep problems following vigorous exercise close to bedtime. So, the most sensible conclusion is to exercise regularly at whatever time fits although, generally, the earlier in the day you do it the better it would be. If late-evening workouts disrupt sleep but late evening is the only free time you have to exercise, moving to less intense exercises such as stretching or gentle yoga may help.

Exercise is also an extremely effective stress management strategy. Stressful events during the day often carry over into sleep in the form of decreased sleep quality and length as well as unwanted dreams. So, effectively managing stress is a critical aspect of how daytime behaviors influence sleep. For specific recommendations on healthy daytime routines and behaviors for managing stress, see Question 39. Regularly applying sleep hygiene recommendations, discussed further in Question 40, is another critical daytime habit for better sleep.

## 39. What are the best ways to get to sleep at night?

It is hours past bedtime and Raquel hasn't slept well for weeks. After fighting the urge to sleep all day, the struggle reverses at night when she feels wide awake. She messages a friend: How do you force yourself to sleep when you know you need it but your body just refuses to go to sleep?

Sleep occurs when it is the ideal time for it (circadian rhythm) and when sleepiness (adenosine) has built up to the point where it cannot be overcome (homeostatic drive). For example, some people struggle to fall asleep despite feeling sleepy because their body clock is naturally delayed (i.e., a night owl). This struggle can be overcome by shifting the body clock or circadian rhythm timing using light exposure, the main way the body determines sleep and wake time. More precisely, 30 minutes of bright light exposure immediately on awakening in the morning—using sunlight or a consumer light box—essentially tricks the brain into concluding the sunrise occurred earlier than it did in reality. This in turn would cause the body to prepare for sleep earlier the next night, making it easier to fall asleep at a more typical time despite a preference to be a night owl.

The first step toward dealing with difficulties falling asleep is understanding what is causing the problem. Some people struggle to fall asleep at night because they have not built up enough sleepiness or adenosine due to napping, sleeping in, or having an inconsistent wake time. In this case, the treatment would mainly focus on keeping a more consistent sleep-wake routine. Question 22 explores the many factors that contribute to sleep-related problems and discusses possible solutions.

But assuming there is no problem related to biological sleep systems, sleep hygiene, or other underlying sleep or medical conditions, then the continuing problem with falling asleep could be due to stress. It is unlikely that there is a one-size-fits-all solution for getting to sleep at night. If we wanted to help Raquel, we might message her back:

Stop trying to sleep—try to relax instead.

As discussed in Question 23, falling asleep is a process that cannot be directly controlled. The more we try to force sleep, the less likely we are to achieve it. But when we relax, such as on the couch before bedtime, sleep comes naturally and sometimes unexpectedly. It is very possible that Raquel's worries about her sleep needs and difficulties are a big source of stress, which in turn triggers more problems falling asleep.

Feeling "stressed" is a complex biological process of emotional, cognitive, and physical arousal. Stress is also on a spectrum, from subtle signs like lip biting or headaches to more extreme sympathetic nervous system activation, which many people call the "fight-or-flight" response. When these survival mechanisms are triggered by stressful situations, physical changes occur that are not compatible with sleep, such as increased heart rate and breathing, elevated body temperature, and increase in brain chemicals that stimulate wakefulness. So, it is important to reduce stress prior to bedtime.

Everyone experiences stress and it can actually be motivating and useful at moderate levels. Jumping into bed without letting go of normal day-to-day stress is likely to cause problems falling asleep. Instead, Raquel might consider keeping a "buffer zone" between her day and the time she gets in bed. This 30- to 60-minute wind-down period of relaxing activities before bedtime cues the brain to prepare for sleep. A consistent routine serves as a cue to the body that it is time for bed, and the longer one has kept this routine the stronger the influence it will have on sleepiness. This is likely the main reason why a warm glass of milk before bed makes some people feel sleepier; it is a comforting tradition that provides relaxing cues to the brain eliciting sleepiness.

Ideally, Raquel would create a highly personalized routine that can be consistently followed every day to condition her brain and body to sleep more regularly. This routine may include taking a warm bath or shower, turning off electronics an hour before bed, reading, playing music, doing light chores, preparing for the next day, meditating, and so on. Productive activities like homework or discussions that have the potential to cause emotional stress should be avoided during this time. Some people find physical or mental relaxation techniques to be useful during their buffer zone.

While the full breadth of relaxation techniques is beyond the scope of this question, the most commonly used physical relaxation strategies focus on decreasing physiological arousal; these include diaphragmatic or "deep" breathing, autogenic training, and progressive muscle relaxation. Whichever relaxation technique is chosen, Raquel should practice a few times a day, five minutes each time, when already relaxed. This will help her learn the skill and associate it with feeling relaxed, which ultimately increases effectiveness. However, she should not practice relaxation exercises in bed, especially with the goal of forcing sleep via relaxation, as this is an example of trying to control sleep. Practicing out of bed is strongly encouraged to avoid associating the bed with wakefulness, such as during the buffer zone or when getting out of bed due to not being able to sleep.

Some people report feeling "tired but wired," meaning they are physically exhausted but mentally highly alert and unable to sleep, often with racing thoughts. Just like the physical stress response, worries or active thoughts delay sleep by turning on the sympathetic nervous system that overpowers sleep systems. Some people attempt to cope with an active mind by focusing their attention on less stressful content, mainly by watching or listening to entertainment like movies or podcasts. By filling their mind with fun diversions, there is no room to focus on serious stressors. People may delay bedtime with this entertainment or attempt to go to sleep with it playing in the background. In spite of the belief that it helps, sleep studies clearly demonstrate that sleeping with music, television, or other entertainment playing ultimately does more harm than good by causing lighter, less refreshing, and more frequently disrupted sleep.

Everyone has general life concerns but we often avoid thinking about these because it doesn't feel good and it takes time from our busy lives. But ignoring these concerns doesn't make them disappear, it simply delays them for a later time when distractions are absent and the mind can wander—in other words, concerns may return when awake in bed or through nightmares. While pleasant imagery exercises can be helpful in filling the mind with relaxing imagery, this temporary relief is not very effective as the mind returns to worries once it is bored with imagery exercises or once the exercises have been completed.

Knowing that we ultimately cannot avoid our problems or worries, Raquel might be encouraged to make time for them during the day. This sort of works like a pressure release valve. By choosing a time that works better to worry and sticking with it, the brain is given an opportunity to address concerns earlier so there's less pressure to address them in bed. Fifteen minutes of daily journaling is one method for offloading concerns. Other individuals find benefit from the use of a "concerns list" for quieting the mind, spending 15 minutes at the same time daily listing all worries and concerns while noting a "first step" for how they might begin addressing each problem.

Whatever the method, it can be helpful to make time to address worries in the early evening, before the buffer zone, so your brain doesn't feel the need to do it in bed. It often takes a week or two of consistently using this strategy before it begins to work because the brain needs to learn that you will follow through with keeping worry time consistent each day. After this time, if worries still arise in bed, it can be useful to reassure oneself with self-talk like: "Thank you for the reminder brain, but I already thought about this problem today and I can think more about it during my scheduled worry time tomorrow. For now, I just want to relax."

Many clinicians also utilize mindfulness techniques to help patients let go of the perceived need to control sleep. Mindfulness meditation has been used to provide relief to those reporting high stress, anxiety, and pain conditions that interfere with sleep. In brief, mindfulness is the prac-tice of noticing and being fully aware of one's present experience without needing to change the experience. The mindfulness attitude of simply being in the moment, moving from a state of doing into a state of being, aligns nicely with the ideal attitude to have at bedtime.

If Raquel continues to struggle to "turn it off" despite the use of these relaxation techniques, she may want to consider counseling support to learn alternative strategies for managing stress. These strategies may include increasing daytime physical activity, using written thought logs to examine and challenge unhelpful beliefs, decreasing caffeine and alcohol consumption, eating whole foods and avoiding highly processed foods, and spiritual or religious engagement. People who delay going to sleep to avoid terrifying, reoccurring nightmares would likely also benefit from professional support. However, if Raquel suspects her thoughts relate to more serious mental health concerns, she may need more in-depth psy-chological treatment. Sleep medications should be used with caution and generally only work well in the short term, as discussed in Question 34. However, other mood-related medications may indirectly improve some sleep difficulties and be taken in the longer term.

## 40. Why don't the sleep hygiene tips I read online work?

Sleep hygiene is a lot like dental hygiene. Dental hygiene, like daily floss-ing and brushing your teeth, is critical for prevention of cavities and good oral health. Sleep hygiene, similarly, describes the habits and behaviors critical for preventing sleep problems. If a painful tooth was the result of a cavity, no amount of dental hygiene is going to brush or floss away the problem. Likewise, sleep hygiene alone cannot treat a sleep problem once it has arisen. Even though we cannot floss away a cavity, we do not disregard or ignore dental hygiene recommendations because we know they keep us healthy and can prevent future problems. Sleep hygiene too is a critical part of prevention that we should not overlook; it is also an important part of treatment.

Sleep hygiene is extremely effective when used in conjunction with sleep treatments like stimulus control, discussed in Question 23. But sleep hygiene alone is not an effective treatment. As discussed in Question 22 for example, while poor sleep hygiene may have played a role in the initial development of insomnia, other factors like conditioned arousal can con-tinue to drive the ongoing sleep disruption regardless of whatever sleep hygiene changes are made. In summary, sleep hygiene tips found online or provided by others are good for prevention but inadequate as a sole treatment for a preexisting sleep problem.

Four general factors that influence sleep should be considered when working on improving sleep hygiene: environmental factors, factors impacting sleepiness (i.e., the homeostatic drive to sleep), the genetic time-of-day body clock preferences, and the stress response. As discussed in more detail in Question 6, the ideal environment for sleep is similar to a cave: dark, quiet, cool, and safe.

Keeping a consistent wake time every day is critical to have a consistent level of sleepiness at bedtime each night. Ideally, avoid sleeping in and keep a fairly consistent bedtime. Napping should also be avoided because, in the same way that snacking before a meal reduces appetite, naps decrease the pressure to fall and stay asleep later in the day. If napping is necessary for safety, such as before driving a long distance, ideally complete the nap at least eight hours before bedtime and limit it to 20–30 minutes.

Checking the time while in bed, though very common, is not recommended. While anxiety about missing the alarm clock can drive clock checking, the outcome can be either positive (e.g., feeling reassured when there is plenty of time left to sleep) or, more commonly, negative (e.g., "here we go again" —angry thoughts increasing alertness, the person feeling pressured to sleep since there is limited time remaining). Instead, consider setting an alarm and placing the phone or clock a bit out of reach. When awakening at night, it may be necessary at first to reassure oneself with self-talk (e.g., "It doesn't matter what time it is, the alarm will let me know when I need to get up, right now I just need to relax.") until the desire to check the time diminishes. Finally, avoid using the snooze feature on the morning alarm, as discussed in Question 42.

Caffeine is one of the most commonly used drugs worldwide due in part to its ability to suppress feelings of sleepiness, as discussed in depth in Question 36. Depending on an individual's tolerance to the drug, caffeine noticeably increases alertness for at least six to eight hours. Although some individuals are able to fall asleep with caffeine active in their systems, their sleep will not be very deep or refreshing, which increases cravings for caffeine the following day. To prevent this, caffeine should be avoided roughly eight hours prior to bedtime—after lunch for most people—and limited to about two servings a day.

Although people vape, dip, and smoke nicotine to relax, it acts as a stimulant increasing wakefulness and disrupting sleep. Nicotine should be avoided before bedtime to the extent that's possible without causing withdrawal cravings that can disrupt sleep. Likewise, although initially relaxing and helpful for falling asleep, alcohol should be avoided because it disrupts the quality of sleep overall, making us feel sleepier and more stressed the following day. Finally, while occasional use of over-the-counter (OTC) sleep aids is not a major cause for concern if limited to a few days, such as during travel to cope with jet lag, repeated use over several weeks should be avoided due to the risk of loss of effectiveness over time and of developing the dangerous belief that sleep is not possible without medicine.

The third factor to be considered for sleep hygiene is the time-of-day body clock preferences, otherwise known as circadian rhythm. As discussed in Question 9, the brain uses environmental cues to regulate the timing of sleep and wakefulness. The strongest cue is from sunlight or blue spectrum light, followed by timing of exercise and meals and environmental temperature, as discussed in Question 38. Given this, it is helpful to avoid LED screens and light bulbs beginning one hour before bedtime and throughout the night (e.g., avoid checking the phone in bed, avoid use of TV at night). Conversely, morning light exposure can reduce grogginess by increasing alertness more rapidly.

Successfully managing emotional stress is the fourth sleep-hygiene consideration. Standard recommendations for stress management include regular physical activity or exercise, limiting alcohol and drugs, engaging in fun and meaningful activities, and spending time with others to avoid isolating oneself. Eating a healthy diet of whole foods like fruits, vegetables, fish, nuts, and olive oil have particular benefits for coping with stress. Other techniques for stress management and preparing for sleep have been reviewed in Question 39.

### 41. Why do people say that using the computer or a smartphone before bed is bad for you?

The translated expression "sleepless night revenge" originated in China and spread across social media around the onset of the COVID-19 pandemic. The behavior now known as "revenge bedtime procrastination" occurs when an individual delays going to sleep—despite knowing that they will suffer the following day from sleep loss —to feel a sense of control or freedom or to enjoy time alone. This behavior may provide a temporary sense of relief and enjoyment, but the sleep loss that follows ultimately increases both physical and emotional stress over the course of the following day. While the choice to delay sleep for more immediate pleasures is unlikely to cause significant harm if used rarely (e.g., New

Year's Eve), it ultimately causes the wide-ranging negative consequences of sleep loss if it is frequent. Bluntly, revenge bedtime procrastination is a habit to be avoided.

Often, this habit is paired with electronics use, like watching movies or shows in bed, reading the news from a tablet or phone, or "doom scrolling" (reading disturbing news or comments) endlessly through social media. Knowing this, clinicians discourage use of electronics before bedtime, partly to decrease their distractions or temptations that delay going to sleep. Light exposure and conditioning, discussed below, are responsible for the typical sleep-hygiene recommendation to avoid using electronics or any screen-based device before bedtime. But more information on sleep hygiene can be seen in Question 40.

As discussed in Question 9, the brain uses cues from the environment to determine sleep and wake times; these environmental cues include sunlight, temperature, and timing of meals and exercise. Throughout human history and our brain's evolution, artificial light (i.e., fire) is usually in the orange-yellow spectrum whereas sunlight is in the white-blue spectrum. Technically many colors make up sunlight, but blue is dominant. However, when we perceive the substantial blue light of modern LED screens or light bulbs, our brains wrongly assume it is sunlight. In response to this artificial sunlight, the brain makes chemical changes that increase daytime alertness. When using LED screens before bedtime, people essentially "trick" their brains into concluding the sun has not set and, as a result, they remain awake longer into the night.

Admittedly, using electronics before bed is calming for many people and being relaxed is essential for falling sleep. However, this relaxation approach is like shooting oneself in the foot—to use a common expression— because it comes with the significant cost of creating more alertness and causing difficulties falling asleep. To avoid this light exposure pitfall but still enjoy some electronics use, a common recommendation is to avoid LED screens (e.g., phone, tablet) and light bulbs beginning one hour before bedtime. Turning off all screens an hour early ensures the brain will begin to perceive darkness and naturally release melatonin to help ease the transition into sleep. Alternatively, many modern phones and screens offer night modes which will automatically dim blue light electrodes from the screen at sundown. The effectiveness of these "night modes" is uncertain; but using the night mode is definitely less effective than turning off electronics outright.

Knowing that light increases alertness, LED screens should also be avoided the entire night. For example, checking one's phone for the time during the night may cause the brain to misperceive a phone screen as the beginning of sunrise, thereby increasing alertness. Conversely, increasing light first thing after awakening can alleviate morning grogginess by increasing alertness rapidly. Opening window shades, turning on overhead lights, and using LED light bulbs with higher blue spectrum light indoors will support morning wakefulness. Morning exercise and showering may further assist in achieving wakefulness.

Conditioning is the final major reason to avoid electronics one hour before bedtime. Simply put, conditioning is the process by which a person becomes trained to behave in a certain way, often through repeatedly pairing certain behaviors with certain outcomes. For example, if someone eats food samples every time they visit a warehouse club store, over time they may become conditioned to feeling hunger simply by driving toward the store. When falling asleep, conditioning can be a friend or a foe depending on how it is used.

When difficulties sleeping last for a week or longer, conditioned arousal may begin to arise as the bed is associated with stress and wakefulness. Discussed in detail in Question 22, conditioned arousal is when people feel more alert and stressed simply by getting into the bed. More subtle forms of conditioning resulting in alertness are likely at play when considering the use of electronics before bedtime— particularly cellular phones.

One could easily make the argument that phones are one of the most stimulating things our brains will encounter. Cellular phones, and the easy Internet access they offer, provide a nearly endless supply of entertainment from throughout human history, including music, books, gaming, videos, stories, poems, pictures, and so on. Most human knowledge is accessible online through the phone. Our phones offer up-to-the-minute news, social media postings, weather updates, and sports information, not to mention direct text, video, and voice messages from loved ones. Over time, the inherently alerting nature of cellular phones is made worse as they are further associated with high stimulation and alertness because of conditioning. Given all this, simply touching our cellular phones undoubtedly lights up the brain's pleasure, reward, and alerting systems.

For many reasons, people struggle with avoiding electronics at night. Ideally, all electronics would be turned off one hour before bedtime. If using the cellphone as an alarm clock or bedside clock makes it difficult to avoid touching it at night, then the person might want to consider using an actual bedside clock. Some report use of the phone's "quiet mode" or "airplane mode" at night to avoid sleep-disturbing notifications. Ideally, the phone should be placed out of reach to reduce the temptation to check it during natural middle-of-the-night awakenings.

The wind-down routine used before getting into bed is the key to successful sleep conditioning. Those who consistently use electronics and screens directly before bedtime train the brain to become more alert and delay sleep, as discussed earlier. Having no consistent routine or bedtime preparation behaviors may lead to worsening of problems as well. So consider turning off all electronics and screens one hour before bedtime, keeping a 30- to 60-minute wind-down period or "buffer zone" between daytime activities and bedtime.

This buffer zone should include relaxing activities that serve as a cue to the body that it is time for bed. Activities during this time should be highly personalized to whatever is most calming for the individual, but they may include yoga, meditation, prayer, listening to music, reading books, using relaxation techniques, small talk, artistic expression, or journaling. To increase conditioning effectiveness, only engage in these activities before bedtime. The longer one keeps this routine the stronger the influence it will have on sleepiness. For more ideas on how to fall asleep easily without the use of electronics, see Question 39.

### 42. Why can't I get out of bed on time, and why do I turn off the alarm without even realizing it?

Most people with difficulties getting out of bed blame this struggle on what scientists call sleep inertia. This is a typical response to awakening which involves feeling physically weak or slow, mental fogginess with difficulty thinking logically, less sensory awareness of the environment, and a strong desire to return to sleep. These symptoms are entirely normal when we first wake up to a degree, but when overly powerful, they may highlight an underlying sleep problem. Difficulty getting out of bed in the morning can be caused by problems with not getting enough sleep, awakening at a time that conflicts with the brain's natural timing preference, or psychological factors like habits, thoughts, and mood.

The transition from sleep to wakefulness is gradual, not immediate. Sleep inertia is the period of time during which the effects of sleep linger and seep into wakefulness. For well-rested, healthy adults with normal circadian rhythms, sleep inertia grogginess will still occur, even following a full night of sleep, and last for around 5–30 minutes. For biological "morning larks" who naturally wake early, full awakening is usually achieved in less than 5 minutes. Alternatively, "night owls," who function best in the evenings, experience longer sleep inertia in the mornings that often last for more than 30 minutes (depending on how early the final awakening occurred).

To a certain degree, getting out of bed is hard for most teenagers due to normal biological changes conflicting with daily obligations. The natural delay in sleep timing occurring during adolescence, causes the tendency towards late bedtimes and late wake times. These trends resemble the sleep timings of genetic "night owls" discussed in depth in Question 9, and play a major role in the struggle with sleep inertia and getting out of bed. When school and other activities require teens to awaken earlier than they are naturally inclined to, sleep inertia grogginess becomes stronger. This contributes to sleep deprivation as teenagers are physically unable to fall asleep until late in the evening but are forced to awaken early for school.

Considering that sleep inertia is inevitable, judging the quality of your sleep based on how you feel when you first awaken is an unfair and inaccurate measurement. Instead, a better measure of sleep quality is how alert or sleepy one feels several hours after awakening. It isn't possible to eliminate sleep inertia but it can be shortened and its impact decreased by increasing bright light exposure as soon as possible following awakening. This technique is discussed further in Question 43.

Other factors must be considered when explaining why some people simply cannot get out of bed, even if they set an alarm and are fully awake. Many psychological factors can drive people to remain in bed, but they are too extensive to review in depth. They include things like a desire to avoid the day and the stressors that come along with it (i.e., avoidance), a preference to "ease into" the day by using the snooze alarm feature a few times (i.e., habit), a desire to put off feared or unpleasant daytime tasks (i.e., procrastination), unhealthy thoughts such as negative predictions of how the day will proceed or how sleep will impact daytime functioning (i.e., cognitive distortions), or feeling low, sluggish, and unconcerned about getting out of bed due to a mood disorder like depression.

Knowing how difficult it can be to get out of bed in the morning, some people rely heavily on their alarm's snooze feature in the hope that a few additional minutes of sleep may help offset sleepiness. Unfortunately, the type of slow-wave sleep that helps us feel restored and refreshed mostly occurs at the beginning of the night and is highly unlikely to occur during a brief morning snooze or nap. Not only does snoozing fail to make us feel more rested, it actually increases and intensifies the unavoidable grogginess of sleep inertia. When multiple early alarms are set prior to the desired final wake time to ease transition into wakefulness, the brain is effectively awake from the moment of the first alarm. So, this strategy ultimately backfires by decreasing overall total sleep and increasing daytime sleepiness.

Many people use the snooze feature, or turn off their alarm altogether, without remembering that they did it. Others insist their alarm clock must be broken because they have no memory of turning it off. In these cases, sleep inertia is to blame once again. When we are first jolted awake by an alarm, our brain is not fully operational as it works to come online and orient itself. During this time, thinking is illogical and disorganized, and the logic of not turning off the alarm or avoiding snoozing is lost. Similar to how we typically forget our frequent but brief middle-of-the-night awakenings, many do not remember turning off their alarms or using the snooze feature because they did not remain awake long enough to form a memory of doing so.

In summary, we should expect some degree of grogginess when we first awaken, but it's best to fight the urge to snooze. As hard as it can be to simply put one's feet on the floor, the sooner one gets out of bed following the alarm, thereby increasing movement and light exposure, the sooner one will overcome sleep inertia. Additional recommendations for awakening successfully and getting out of bed on time are addressed in the next question.

### 43. How can I train myself to wake up earlier and remain awake and alert?

In an online forum, a college freshman posted a request for "sleep hacks" to help with getting out of bed early and remaining awake in morning class. While most replies focused on use of caffeine, a more comprehensive recipe for success could be summarized as: People who awaken more easily and feel more alert throughout the day are those who get 1) enough, 2) good quality, and 3) consistent sleep, apart from having 4) healthy sleep habits and 5) realistic expectations of sleep.

When teenagers get less than 8–10 hours of sleep, and when adults receive less than 7–8 hours, awakening and maintaining daytime alertness becomes much more difficult. Sleep loss also increases sleep inertia, as discussed in Question 42, which makes it harder to wake up and remain alert. At least as important as length, however, is the quality of sleep. Those who fall asleep initially in about 15–20 minutes, and perhaps awaken briefly several times during the night but otherwise remain asleep, typically have good quality sleep. Underlying disorders that disrupt sleep quality, like nightmares or narcolepsy, can also contribute to problems with waking, but those require clinical assessment.

The old adage "you snooze, you lose" can be taken quite literally with regard to sleep, because use of the alarm's snooze feature is associated with losing more sleep. It's best to set the alarm for the latest possible wake time while still having enough time to prepare for the day. This way, total sleep time can be maximized over time. Keeping a consistent wake time on both weekdays and weekends, regardless of how much sleep occurred the night before, and avoiding sleeping in helps to synchronize the body clock, increase daytime alertness and, ultimately, improve nighttime sleep.

Some blame their difficulties with awakening on the alarm itself and ask, "which is the best alarm clock to guarantee I wake up?" Many creative alarm solutions have been marketed: a clock that launches puzzle pieces around the room that must be reassembled to silence the alarm; a sunrise light simulator; an app that requires completion of a math problem; a vibrating bed pad; and (amusingly) a paper shredder alarm that destroys the sleeper's money if ignored. No major research has compared these products so the best alarm clock is whatever works for you. Based on user reports, alarms requiring more brain processing to silence the alarm—such as solving a math problem or getting out of bed to complete a physical task—tend to be most successful. Placing the alarm clock further away, which requires getting out of bed to silence it, can also assist with awakening.

Following healthy sleep habits, known as sleep hygiene and discussed in Question 40, is an important aspect of awakening more easily and feeling more refreshed in the daytime. Ideally, it is best to avoid naps and aim for a regular bedtime on most days. If mood difficulties like depression or high stress are interfering with sleep, it's important to address these concerns. Unrealistic expectations and stressful thoughts about sleep (e.g., "If I feel sleepy when I first wake up, it means I need more sleep") may need to be challenged. Improvements are most likely to occur when all these strategies are combined.

Although one can "train" oneself to awaken early using the behavioral strategies discussed, we are somewhat limited by our unalterable genetics, which determine when we naturally prefer to fall asleep and awaken (see Question 9). Some people struggle to wake up early because they are fighting against their natural sleep-timing preference. So, despite the use of behavioral strategies, people who identify as "night owls" tend to experience more severe morning grogginess even if they are regularly getting good quality sleep. In this case, it is important to have realistic expectations and know that sleep inertia is normal and time-bound, albeit stronger for night owls, and usually less disabling than people believe it to be.

Although genetic preferences for sleep timing cannot be changed, the circadian rhythm can be temporarily altered using light. In essence, the circadian rhythm can be tricked into thinking it is a different time of day than the actual clock time. For people who struggle with getting out of bed in the morning due to a biological night preference, adjusting light exposure and timing can shift the body clock. Bright light in the morning shifts the body clock forward, as if it were later in the day than it really is, which increases morning alertness and assists in awakening more rapidly. Conversely, for "morning larks" who struggle with remaining awake in the evenings or awakening too early in the mornings, evening bright light shifts the body clock backward, as if it were earlier in the day. This tends to delay falling asleep to a more typical time and decreases early morning awakenings.

For people who struggle with getting out of bed due to circadian factors, it helps to increase bright morning light exposure as soon as possible after awakening. While opening window shades and turning on all the room lights can help, most research finds maximum benefits from either one hour outside in bright sunlight or 30 minutes in front of a light box (i.e., consumer light boxes with full spectrum 10,000 lux light are easily available online and often used to treat seasonal mood difficulties). Whatever method is chosen, these strategies are known to increase alertness, improve mood, assist in remaining awake and alert, and help with falling asleep one to two hours earlier the following night.

Caffeine can also be useful for individuals who struggle to get out of bed, as long as it is not overused and it is stopped at least eight hours prior to bedtime. Everyone naturally experiences a midafternoon dip in energy after lunchtime. Rather than napping or turning to caffeine during this time, which runs the risk of impairing sleep the following night, a more effective approach would be increasing bright light exposure and engaging in light physical activity in the afternoon. For example, a brisk outdoor walk after lunch can provide the alerting boost needed to remain awake and alert for the remainder of the day.

## 44. Is there anything I can do to stop having bad dreams?

About 90 percent of the population experiences nightmares about once a month, which is normal and does not require treatment. Some scientists even argue that bad dreams are helpful because they allow us to role-play different solutions to survive potentially stressful situations. But if bad dreams occur at least a few times a week, something may need to be done.

The first step is to determine what caused the dreams. Nightmares most often result from higher daytime stress, not getting enough sleep, and frequent sleep disruption, but bad dreams also cause these problems to worsen over time. Some people hope to avoid the suffering of nightmares by delaying bedtime for as long as possible. Sadly, avoiding sleep to avoid nightmares causes greater daytime stress and sleep deprivation, both of which increase nightmares. So, breaking this vicious cycle most effectively usually involves simultaneously addressing all contributing factors—mental health, sleep quality and quantity, and other factors interfering with sleep and dream quality.

Mental health disorders, particularly anxiety and depression, are highly associated with nightmares. Approximately 88 percent of people with post-traumatic stress disorder (PTSD) experience nightmares regularly. So, seeking treatment for underlying mental health problems is a key component of improving dreams. Likewise, using healthy stress management techniques to offload physical and emotional stress prior to bedtime is recommended, such as by journaling, diaphragmatic "deep" breathing, and regular physical activity.

In addition to addressing emotional stress, a second critical component of eliminating bad dreams is to improve sleep quality and to sleep no less than seven hours every night. As discussed in Question 23 in greater detail, cognitive behavioral therapy for insomnia (CBT-I) is a psychological treatment for difficulties falling and staying asleep that works extremely effectively. Using research-based techniques, CBT-I essentially retrains the brain to sleep naturally using a variety of strategies— stimulus control, sleep hygiene, sleep efficiency training, stress management, challenging unhelpful thinking, measured exposure to avoided nightmare content, and mindfulness. Other psychological therapies for nightmares, but with much more limited research, include rescripting therapy, sleep dynamic therapy, systematic desensitization, and guided imagery with hypnosis.

One of the most frequently researched treatments for nightmares is a psychological intervention called imagery rehearsal therapy (IRT). In brief, IRT works by having people repeatedly imagine a new dream script multiple times daily over several weeks in order to change the content of their dreams into something more bearable, neutral, or positive. Just as a full day spent playing videogames can result in a night full of vivid, videogame-like dreams, a day spent frequently imagining or rehearsing pleasant dream imagery can influence the content of dreams that night. Perhaps inspired by this parallel to gaming, scientists today are looking at the use of virtual reality to provide computer-generated sights and sounds for individuals who struggle to produce mental imagery during IRT dream rehearsal.

For people who complete IRT by working with a licensed clinician, the benefits can be dramatic. Variations of IRT in multiple studies have found it decreases nightmare frequency and intensity, reduces symptoms of depression, anxiety, and fear of sleep, and decreases the symptoms and severity of PTSD in those with PTSD-related nightmares. Sometimes nightmares are eliminated entirely, with the benefits enduring long term. Sleep quality is also improved, with more rapid sleep onset and decreased nighttime disruption as well as increased total sleep time. For an example of IRT in action, see Case Study 3, "A Better-Ending Story."

The third and final factor contributing to nightmares is anything that interferes with normal biological control of sleep and dream quality. This includes any untreated sleep disorders, like sleep-related breathing disorders, which cause frequent awakenings and chronic sleep deprivation. Attending to unaddressed medical issues that impact sleep (e.g., asthma, diabetes, chronic obstructive pulmonary disease) is another important aspect of reducing unwanted dreams.

When experiencing disrupted sleep due to nightmares, some people turn to over-the-counter (OTC) sleep aids. Melatonin is a popular OTC choice for sleep; however, its most common side effect is vivid dreams or nightmares. Given this, those experiencing nightmares should avoid melatonin and other medications that are known to cause nightmares, including many sleep aids, antidepressants, and beta blockers. Caffeine, alcohol, nicotine, and recreational drugs should also be avoided.

Prazosin is a medication for high blood pressure that is often used to reduce nightmare frequency, nighttime awakenings, and PTSD severity. Some studies have called into question its effectiveness within certain subpopulations, but many have unquestionably found benefit from it in reducing nightmares as well as in improving sleep quality and quantity. Further research would clarify who is most likely to benefit from prazosin but it is important to recognize that even if it is effective, nightmares often return once the medication is stopped. Other medications are sometimes used for nightmare treatment clinically but have little to no research data to back them up; these include clonidine, trazodone, topiramate, gabapentin, and antipsychotics.

Compared to taking medicine alone (i.e., prazosin), IRT is more effective and has fewer side effects. When IRT is combined with CBT-I, the benefits easily surpass those of medications and people report even fewer nightmares, less awakenings, and lower PTSD severity. The additional benefits likely arise because CBT-I improves sleep quality, which in turn decreases nightmare occurrence.

Recent research suggests that galantamine, a dementia medication, may also increase lucid dreaming frequency. As discussed in Question 11, lucid dreaming can be one route of eliminating nightmares, so galantamine may someday be used in conjunction with lucid dreaming interventions. How this might compare to IRT will be a critical question to answer.

When experiencing frequent bad dreams, many people turn to alcohol, nicotine, cannabis, recreational drugs, or afternoon caffeine to cope. However, as reviewed in Questions 35 and 36, each of these is known to disrupt normal sleep and dreaming patterns and may trigger nightmares. While potentially relaxing and seemingly helpful initially, these substances are biologically stressful and alerting, ultimately causing more dream and sleep disruption in the long term. Ironically, our attempts at self-medicating away nightmares are often the driving factor in bringing them back.

# Case Studies

## 1. RUNNING ON EMPTY

Anja's best friend Julia was in tears as she exclaimed, "I can't believe you didn't show up. It was my birthday. What kind of friend are you?" Anja begged her not to take it personally. "I had study group for Chem, and it just slipped my mind. Look, it's not about you, Julia. I'm just super busy."

Anja's sister had warned her that if she wanted to get into college, senior year would be like this. Essays for English and History were due every Friday. Chemistry was impossible, and she'd be lucky to earn a C in it. The worst was Spanish—no matter how hard Anja drilled, she couldn't remember the vocabulary. Swim team was from 4:00 to 6:00 p.m., and at night there was homework and online study group, leaving only a few hours after 11:00 p.m. to catch up with friends. On Saturdays and Sundays, Anja taught children to swim at the local pool. Colleges expect to see community service, she reminded herself, and she needed the money.

The night Anja screamed at her parents, they began to worry. They had heard her talking to her friends at 2:00 a.m. and told her she'd have to get to bed earlier. "You've been grumpy," they added, "and you're always yawning. What's wrong?" But Anja insisted she was just fine, she wasn't feeling tired, and she always caught up on sleep over the weekend anyway. "I'm not a child anymore! I don't need as much sleep as I used to. And I have a right to have friends, don't I?" she shouted.

That Thursday began like most days, except Anja figured that getting up a little earlier at 6:00 a.m. to review would give her a handle on her

Spanish. While driving to school, she stopped off for a double espresso, which would prop her up until noon. Then she had an energy drink at lunch, although that sometimes made her jittery and made it hard to concentrate. On the drive back home from swim practice, she began plotting out the evening hour by hour. She was thinking she might need to stop for another coffee to make it through that evening's study session. The next thing she knew, she felt her head hit the steering wheel. The car was up on the sidewalk, and she had smashed into a streetlamp. She had fallen asleep. Fortunately, she was okay, just very shaken. But she would have to explain the dent to her parents.

The next day, Anja's parents drove her to their family doctor, who did a quick physical exam, ordered a blood test, pulled out a clipboard, and began asking Anja about her schedule. "Let's see," the doctor said, "one or two double espressos, that's 200–300 mg of caffeine, plus around 160 mg from the energy drink." She looked up from the clipboard, adding, "And four hours of sleep on school nights. Anja, you need to take better care of yourself." "I catch up on Sundays," replied Anja, sheepishly. The doctor continued her questioning, learning that Anja had been irritable with her friends, that she was increasingly forgetful, and that she was having trouble concentrating in classes. Anja denied feeling depressed but admitted she was worried about college.

Later, Anja's doctor conveyed her diagnosis. "There's nothing wrong with your blood, your heart, or your thyroid. This is a case of chronic stress and exhaustion. And you are going to have to do something about it right away or the next time in the car, you may not be so lucky." The doctor advised Anja to get nine hours of sleep a night. She handed her a list of caffeine quantities in coffee and energy drinks and suggested she cut back to no more than one cup of coffee in the morning. Then she spoke with Anja's parents. "You all need to have a talk. About stress, about sleep, about letting go of some of Anja's activities."

Anja and her parents worked out a plan. To start with, there would be no driving until she was getting at least eight hours of sleep a night. She'd work toward an 11:00 p.m. bedtime and ending phone calls by 10:00 p.m. Her school counselor helped her get a tutor for Chemistry and Spanish and some support with college applications. Anja found it hard to cut back on caffeine for the first two weeks; her head ached and she felt sleepy in the afternoons, but she tried to restrict her coffee to the mornings. She reduced her job hours to one day a week. She accepted that everyone struggles with stress and overwork sometimes, but she promised herself she would try to put her friends, her family, and her health first. She hoped she'd never let things get that far again.

### Analysis

The National Sleep Foundation recommends that for mental and physical health, teens aged 14–17 years should get between 8 and 10 hours of sleep over each 24-hour period. Unfortunately, recent studies show that nightly hours of sleep decline through the teen years and that by the end of high school, fewer than 25 percent of students get sufficient sleep. Insufficient sleep syndrome is a serious and chronic state of sleep deprivation in which people routinely get fewer than the recommended number of hours of sleep. Rather than being caused by an inability to sleep, insufficient sleep is caused by not making sleep a high priority. Among teens, this is typically due to heavy school and work demands and late-night social activities.

Like Anja, some people get accustomed to a chronic state of fatigue due to sleep deprivation and are unaware of its impact on their mood and functioning. The impact of sleep loss is harder on the teenage brain than on the adult brain, and it includes problems in school, difficulty paying attention, fatigue, depression, irritability, and anxiety. However, both teens and adults with insufficient sleep have a higher risk of accidents and medical problems.

Caffeine can temporarily conceal the body's sleepiness, but eventually sleepiness will catch up. Sleeping in over the weekends feels better but does not prevent the consequences of sleep deprivation and irregular sleep patterns. The American Academy of Pediatrics recommends that young people restrict caffeine to 100 mg a day—no more than a medium-size cup of coffee. Anja was fortunate to have a supportive family who guided her in her efforts to reduce her work hours, embrace more realistic school-work expectations, scale back on caffeine consumption, and maintain consistent bedtimes. Symptoms of insufficient and irregular sleep typically improve after about two weeks of getting enough sleep.

### 2. UP ALL NIGHT WITH NEMESIS DAWN

"Well, at least it's a great way to learn geography," joked Sebastian, who by tenth grade had formed a tight online gaming group with Leo in Finland, Wang Lei in China, and Adam in Israel. Sebastian had been introduced to Nemesis Dawn by his friends in middle school. They'd begin new quests after school around 4:00 p.m., then break for dinner and homework and connect up again later to play late into the night. He loved many online games, but he was most skilled at this one.

These late-night sessions were his favorites. In fact, he had always been the kind of person who preferred going to sleep later than most and sleeping in late. When it came to schoolwork, he noticed he seemed to concentrate best and hit peak mental performance long after dinner. But waking at 6:30 a.m. for 8:00 a.m. school felt like torture. He yawned through his morning classes and could barely pay attention. He wished that the school would start realizing that teens are different from adults and start classes later in the morning. His parents didn't approve of his late hours, but they figured that he had a "night owl" personality like his dad, who also preferred to work at night. Sebastian's parents concluded that he generally got his schoolwork done and they would just do their best to get him to school on time.

As Sebastian's online gaming proficiency grew throughout middle school, he joined Nemesis Dawn Universal, the international version. By then he was already ranked within the top 100 in the United States, and he figured that if he kept practicing, the world leader's board might be within reach. During the summer break before tenth grade, he played nearly every day, making friends around the world and playing late into the night until his typical 4:00 a.m. bedtime.

The serious problems started when school resumed in the fall. Sebastian set the alarm for 6:30 a.m. each morning but would repeatedly hit the snooze button—sometimes without even realizing it—and continue sleeping. He even tried leaving his phone at the other side of the room to force himself to get out of bed to turn off the alarm. His mother would enter his bedroom at 7:00 a.m. and shake him awake, bringing his clothing to him and driving him to school. He tried napping in the afternoon, but no matter how sleepy he felt, he couldn't doze.

Sebastian's parents became tired of dragging him to school and wanted him to stop isolating himself in his bedroom with the computer. Arguing with them nearly every day, Sebastian hated that no one seemed to understand he was as serious about Nemesis Dawn as any athlete would be about their sport. Finally, Sebastian's parents forbade him to play after 10:00 p.m., which made him feel miserable. His gaming partners were his best friends, and Nemesis Dawn was the only part of his life that was working out. So, he started playing secretly on his smartphone at night.

Sebastian's grades began to drop. He already had more tardy marks and absences by October than what was permitted for the semester. Finally, he fell asleep in a morning class and was placed on detention. The assistant principal phoned his parents and threatened suspension for truancy unless Sebastian immediately began attending his morning classes regularly.

Worried that Sebastian could be expelled, his family consulted a sleep specialist who identified his circadian sleep disorder. The specialist explained that around 15 percent of people have a lifelong physical tendency to fall asleep and wake up two or more hours later than most people, and Sebastian had probably inherited this tendency from his father. When this trait causes chronic problems in daily work, school, and socializing, it's called delayed sleep-wake phase disorder (DSWPD). The sleep specialist also helped Sebastian confront the consequences of his all-night gaming. By scaling back his middle-of-the-night gameplay, he would reduce his gaming but could continue to enjoy the benefits it brought to him, such as feeling successful and being online with friends, and he could begin to gain back a normal life.

Together, they set a bedtime goal of 11:00 p.m. and instituted chronotherapy treatment. At the start of treatment his habitual bedtime was 4 a.m. For chronotherapy, Sebastian was guided to intentionally delay going to sleep two hours later each nights for almost 10 days, shifting his sleep time forward two hours each night until he was able to get to sleep by the goal bedtime of 11 p.m.. For the first two weeks, he was even more tired than usual. Sebastian's family met with his assistant principal and discussed how to help transition him back to a regular school day. The school agreed to reschedule Sebastian's early morning lab class for the late afternoon, which made on-time arrival a little easier.

### Analysis

DSWPD is most common during adolescence, when young people's internal clocks tend to shift naturally to favor later bedtimes and later wake times. Like his father, Sebastian could be called a night owl, as he naturally functions at his best late in the day and at night. In addition to his natural late-sleep preference, Sebastian fell into a pattern of late-night gaming, losing his normal circadian rhythm of nighttime sleep and daytime activity, with serious consequences.

Many people with DSWPD benefit from keeping consistent sleep-wake times, chronotherapy treatment as described earlier, increasing early morning exposure to sunlight or artificial lights in the frequencies of sunlight, and changing work and school schedules to reduce morning responsibilities. Sebastian and his parents will need to address his persistence with late-night gaming despite the negative consequences to his academic and family life; they will also need to consider whether he might need further professional support to help him reduce the time spent on videogames.

Finally, Sebastian attends a high school with an 8:00 a.m. start time. While this can be challenging for most teens, early morning start times can particularly jeopardize school performance for someone with DSWPD.

Unfortunately, although adults can often shift their work times to accommodate their circadian rhythm preference, teens can rarely control their daily school schedule. A movement advocating for later school start times during adolescence is now gaining international momentum. Proponents say school experiments that moved daily start times to 8:30 a.m. or later led to students getting more sleep, reduced absenteeism, improved mental and physical health, decreased motor vehicle accidents, and better grades and higher standardized test scores.

## 3. A BETTER-ENDING STORY

Maya finally knew what it meant when people said, "Now I've seen something I can't unsee." Three weeks earlier, she and her friend Raul were driving on a quiet highway when a deer sprang out of the forest, recoiled as it saw their car, and then bounded across the road toward an oncoming motorcycle. They watched in horror as the motorcycle swerved around the deer, slid out, and threw its rider off the road. Maya, a 19-year-old nursing student with a CPR (cardiopulmonary resuscitation) certification, instructed Raul to park, call 911, and set up warning flares for other drivers.

Safe from traffic, she approached the unconscious victim and remembered her CPR basics: checking for pulse while watching for breathing effort, doing chest compression, opening and clearing the airway, and then applying rescue breaths. Ten minutes later, the emergency paramedics arrived and took over. Maya and Raul observed them examining the man's injuries, using equipment to stimulate his heart, and carrying him off on a stretcher. Before speeding off in the ambulance, one of the paramedics turned to Maya. "I'm sorry," he said. "You did everything you could. But I'm afraid it wasn't enough."

Each night afterward, it was as if she were watching a slow-motion replay of the accident in her nightmares: the deer looking into their eyes, the sound of the motorcycle swerving, the man sliding off the road, the smells of gasoline and blood, the struggle against fatigue to continue CPR. But the worst part of the nightmare was the paramedic saying to her, "It wasn't enough." Then she'd wake up crying, sweating, and breathing heavily, with her heart pounding. At those moments she would feel guilty that she must have made a mistake, telling herself, "If I can't even save a life using CPR, what kind of nurse am I? I am a failure."

During the day, her mind could not shake the details. What did the paramedic mean when he said "it wasn't enough?" Did she omit a step? If she had done something differently, could she have saved the man's life?

After a week, she was so scared of the nightmare she didn't want to go to sleep. She'd watch videos until after midnight, hoping that if she were totally exhausted, she'd sleep without dreams. Her friend recommended she try some melatonin pills to help her relax at night, but the nightmares persisted. After three weeks, she concluded she didn't belong in nursing school if she couldn't handle an emergency.

Finally, Maya approached one of her nursing professors, explaining that she had witnessed an accident and wished to review the details. After reassuring Maya that she had acted responsibly in the situation, her professor was surprised when Maya began to sob. Maya told her about the nightmares and her self-doubts. Her professor smiled. "You will make a wonderful nurse, Maya. You were compassionate and you held your head together in an emergency. But you'll learn that this is part of being a health professional. Sometimes even when you do everything you can, you can't save a patient. Can I help you make an appointment with a student services counselor for some help with those nightmares?"

Since the nightmares were the most troubling part of the accident, Maya's eventual counselor introduced her to imagery rehearsal therapy (IRT), a treatment to reduce the intensity and frequency of nightmares. Maya understood that nightmares become a learned habit over time, sort of as if the brain is stuck playing the same song on a broken record. Daytime stress causes nightmares, which disrupt sleep and cause increasing daytime stress, snowballing into more and more nightmares. She was also taught about how daytime imagery can influence nighttime dream imagery; for example, watching horror film imagery before bedtime may increase the risks of having nightmares in some people. With this new knowledge, her counselor asked Maya to change her nightmare "in any way you wish" by imagining a new, pleasant dream.

She was encouraged to write down this new dream, as if she were a reporter on the scene, using as much sensory information as possible—what she would hear, smell, taste, feel, and so forth. Maya started, "So I'm driving my car again with Raul, but this time it is daytime, and I can feel the warm sun on my left side. I hear Raul singing his favorite song while I'm sipping on my cool, sparkling water. I can smell the salty sea air drifting through our open windows as the oceanside peaks just over the horizon." In the new dream, she goes on to describe the specific steps in building a fire near the shoreline. As the sun sets, the best friends laugh and sing together near the cozy campfire, eventually lulled into peaceful sleep by the gentle sway of their shared hammock.

Maya made time to sit calmly, three times a day for five minutes each time, including right before bedtime, focusing her imagination only on the new dream, with as much detail as possible. Although she only occasionally dreamed this new dream, within three weeks she noticed the nightmares were less frequent and less intense. After two months of continued imagery practice, the nightmares stopped altogether, and she slept through the night peacefully. She no longer needed to practice the new dream because she had successfully changed the song on the record and broken her nightmare habit. Maya spoke to the counselor a few more times about her reaction to the accident and what it had taught her about herself. Later that year, she noticed that sometimes, when she was under a lot of stress at school, the bad version of the nightmare would return for a night or two, but when she'd wake up she would place her feet on the floor, focusing on the physical sensations of her carpet on her toes and the smell of her lavender diffuser, reminding herself that although the past cannot be changed she can make a better future for others by striving to be the best nurse possible.

### Analysis

Sleep is commonly disturbed by distressing dreams that replay traumatic events, especially those in which one has little control, such as a motor vehicle accident, violence, or a natural disaster. Because Maya has experienced these for less than a month, Maya's experience would probably be diagnosed as "nightmare disorder, acute." Her anxiety, her preoccupation with details of the event, and her irrational self-blame for the outcome of the accident despite having done everything right are also common symptoms of post-traumatic stress, which, if it continues and worsens, could eventually be diagnosed as post-traumatic stress disorder.

Maya was fortunate to have the sympathetic ear of her professor, who reassured her that she did the right thing and that her emotional reaction was normal and understandable. Many of those who suffer from nightmares try unsuccessfully to prevent them by delaying sleep or avoiding dreams using drugs or alcohol, which neither prevent nightmares nor help sleep (see Questions 34 and 35). Although melatonin can sometimes help a person fall asleep, it is a relatively weak sleep aid with vivid dreams being a known side effect that can intensify nightmares. Which is to say, there is probably more harm than good in using melatonin in Maya's situation.

Imagery rehearsal techniques (see Question 44) help people gain control over nightmare imagery by focusing on pleasant, less-disturbing images, by rescripting the outcome of the nightmare story, and sometimes by practicing relaxation or meditation approaches prior to bedtime. Often, once the nightmares subside, sleep and emotional regulation improve, decreasing anxiety and stress related to the disturbing event.

## 4. THERE'S A BIG BEAR IN THE TENT

During his second camping trip of the summer, 13-year-old Darrius lay awake listening to the chatter in nearby tents, feeling truly miserable. Everyone else was sharing laughs in the big shelters, while he had to sleep alone in the single tent—an outcast for the crime of snoring. Even so, the other kids still complained they could hear the snorting and coughing from where Darrius slept at the far edge of their campsite. While he enjoyed being popular, he hated his nickname "Darrius Bearius" when others teased him about his weight and nightly "roaring." He was tired in general and dragged himself through the camp activities.

When he returned to school in the fall, Darrius's snoring continued and his daytime sleepiness made it hard to pay attention to teachers or do schoolwork. When it was time for his annual physical, Darrius and his father told the doctor about his snoring, which had increased over the summer. The doctor checked his throat and examined the size and shape of his head and neck. The tonsil glands at the rear of his throat were very large. Darrius was also allergic to several trees and grasses, so he was encouraged to begin taking allergy medication. His doctor said the congestion from the allergies led him to breathe through his mouth which, together with the large tonsils, contributed to the snoring.

Darrius's doctor also informed them that snoring is one sign of obstructive sleep apnea (OSA), which causes sleep problems and daytime sleepiness. She explained that OSA involves momentary pauses in airflow during sleep despite efforts to breathe. She gave Darrius a special adolescent-and-child version of a checklist called the STOP-BANG that included eight risk factors for OSA in teens. Darrius checked off that he snores loudly, that he is sleepy during the daytime, that others have told him he seems to stop breathing at times during sleep, that he was having academic problems, and that he is male. The doctor confirmed one more item—that Darrius's weight for his height was in the overweight range. His STOP-BANG score, 6 out of 8, suggested that Darrius had high risk for sleep apnea. An overnight sleep study would be the next step to confirm the diagnosis, so Darrius left the office with a referral to a local sleep lab.

On the evening of the sleep study, Darrius and his father arrived at the sleep lab after dinner. He was nervous and didn't know what to expect, so he was surprised that the lab looked like a small hotel room, with a bed for Darrius and a sleeping cot for his dad. Having his dad there was reassuring. When it was close to Darrius's bedtime, the sleep technician placed sensors on his head, body, and legs to measure his brain waves, heart function, and muscle and eye movements; an elastic belt was attached around his chest and his stomach to measure breathing, and a finger clip was used to measure the oxygen levels in his blood. There was also a microphone to detect snoring and another microphone to be used if Darrius had any questions for the technician next door, such as for assistance getting to the bathroom during the night. Darrius eventually went to sleep until the next morning, when the technician arrived to detach the sensors so Darrius could head home.

Darrius and his father had a follow-up visit with the sleep physician a week later. Darrius was not surprised to learn he had snored loudly. He was more surprised to learn that he had OSA, with more than 10 apneas an hour associated with a drop in his blood oxygen and frequent episodes of waking throughout the night. Although Darrius spent nine hours in bed each night, he had very little deep, restful sleep. This explained his sleepiness throughout the day. The physician's first recommendation was that Darrius get surgery to remove his tonsils. Explaining that excessive weight also increases the severity of apnea, she also strongly recommended that Darrius increase his daily exercise and work with a nutritionist to find ways to eat healthier.

A month later, Darrius stayed overnight at the hospital for the tonsillectomy. His throat was sore for a week afterward, but he was able to go back to school. At a follow-up sleep study three months after his tonsillectomy, Darrius's sleep looked nearly normal, with almost no apneas and only occasional, light snoring. He felt more rested in the morning, and he was able to concentrate much better in class. Losing weight was a challenge, but as deep sleep became more consistent every night, Darrius had more energy to take up cycling.

### Analysis

OSA (see Question 25) results when the tissues in the mouth and throat block the airways during sleep, creating pauses in breathing, snoring, gasping, and frequent waking. Although the sufferer may appear to be getting enough sleep, breathing struggles cause interrupted, nonrestful sleep that negatively affects daytime schoolwork and other activities. Because sleep problems are known to be common in teens, OSA symptoms often go unnoticed. OSA is more common among males and risk is highest among teens with obesity and enlarged adenoids or tonsils. Darrius had many years of snoring prior to his diagnosis. Occasional snoring is normal, but nightly loud snoring accompanied by pauses in breathing during sleep, like Darrius experienced, should be addressed with a doctor. Untreated OSA is a severe concern for teens, increasing risk for high blood pressure, heart problems, and weight gain in later years.

In some teens, OSA improves with surgical removal of enlarged tonsils and adenoids. The most common treatment for OSA among adults is the continuous positive airway pressure (CPAP) machine, a breathing device that provides pressurized room air through a tube into a mask over the nose, mouth, or both. This consistent flow of air throughout the night holds open the airway, normalizing breathing and, consequently, decreasing sleep disruption. Some people find the CPAP awkward or uncomfortable at first. When feeling embarrassed to use the mask around friends, it helps to practice describing sleep apnea to friends and explaining how the CPAP helps with breathing and daytime functioning. Finally, because excess body fat can enlarge the soft tissues of the throat and create a barrier to breathing, exercise and weight loss efforts are important.

## 5. WORRIES ABOUT WORRYING

Jamie, a high school senior, had a little plaque on her bedroom wall that said, "when I have nothing to worry about, I worry about that!" She used to think this was funny, but of late it felt sadly true. Mostly, she was worrying about her 70-year-old grandmother, Nanna, who had broken her hip. Adding to her worries were her concerns about her own sleep—she could barely remember what a good night's sleep felt like.

After Nanna returned home from the hospital, Nanna's church friends helped with daytime errands while Jamie was at school, and Jamie moved into Nanna's apartment to assist at night. Nanna was like a second mother to Jamie, and Jamie wanted to help. Nanna would ring a bell at night if she needed pain medicine or needed to get to the bathroom. Over time, Nanna started feeling better and no longer woke Jamie, but Jamie would still lie awake in her bedroom. Sometimes she'd get out of bed and stand at Nanna's bedroom door, listening for her breathing, afraid Nanna might fall out of bed or even die.

After three months, Nanna could walk again and told Jamie she could return home to her mother. But back at home, it was as if Jamie had forgotten how to sleep. She would toss and turn in bed, thinking about Nanna all alone in her apartment. She'd worry about money and school and then she would pull out her phone to calculate her budget or text friends. As the sleepless hours continued, sometimes she'd watch TV and fall asleep on the couch in the living room, but when she'd return to bed, she'd be wide awake again.

Jamie tried everything—counting sheep, meditation apps—but even if she did fall asleep, she'd wake up again, realizing that only a couple of hours had passed. She tried some "sleep-aid" allergy medicine that helped briefly but caused a hangover or drowsiness the next morning that she would cope with by drinking coffee all day. She was certain she was getting no more than three hours of sleep a night, and the only thing that helped a little was taking naps after school. Eventually, she started to consider dropping out.

Jamie asked her family doctor for a sleep medication. Her doctor said that while there were some medications that could temporarily help her sleep, the best long-term treatment would be cognitive behavioral therapy for insomnia (CBT-I), a proven approach that would help her body re-learn to sleep normally. Jamie was disappointed not to leave with a sleep medication, but she agreed to give CBT-I a try.

After working with a therapist for two months doing CBT-I, Jamie reported to her doctor, "I think I might be on my way to getting my sleep back!" She described how treatment started and progressed. After two weeks of tracking sleep, naps, time in bed, mood, and coffee, she learned about natural daily sleep functions in the brain and explored how her sleep problems began. She became aware that providing nighttime care at Nanna's had disrupted her familiar sleep patterns and trained her to remain on high alert and vigilant at night, which she described as "sleeping with one eye open."

Like her plaque said, Jamie was prone to worry. Nanna's hip fracture triggered her fears, which were made worse by her anxious concerns about how her lack of sleep was affecting her own health. Eventually, she began to worry about the worries themselves, like how her racing mind prevented her from falling asleep. In treatment, Jamie realized that many of the things she had done to improve her sleep or cope with its loss—like distracting herself with her phone at bedtime, taking allergy medications, drinking coffee, and taking long afternoon naps—were interfering with her body's natural ability to compensate for the lost sleep.

Jamie's treatment started with making lifestyle changes that promote good sleep, known as sleep hygiene. She then learned about stimulus control, guidelines that would help her body associate her bed with sleep rather than wakefulness, such as refraining from using her smartphone or doing schoolwork in bed. Although she knew it would be difficult, she followed the recommendation to stop napping. She learned that napping helped in the short term to compensate for her sleepiness but hurt in the long term by reducing the likelihood of her falling or staying asleep in the evening. She also learned to limit wakefulness in bed by setting a clear bedtime and wake time for each night, which ultimately increases the percentage of time in bed that one is sleeping.

Finally, Jamie learned some practical ways to manage her worrying. Every day before dinner, she would write down a list of her worries, along with one specific first step to deal with the worry, so she was less likely to bring her worries to bed. What may have helped the most, she reflected, was a long talk with Nanna. Nanna reminded her that no one lives forever and that someday Jamie would have to let go of her, but that for now, with Jamie's help, she was all healed up.

### Analysis

Insomnia, a sleep problem involving difficulty falling or staying asleep, is one of the most common sleep problems faced by teens. Although it has many causes, a primary cause is stress. To learn about Jamie's insomnia, her therapist reviewed her sleep diary and did a careful interview, learning about the four factors that cause insomnia, including the 3 Ps—predisposing, precipitating, and perpetuating factors—and conditioned arousal (see Question 22). Predisposing factors are personality or long-lasting medical factors that make it more likely that one will have sleep problems—in Jamie's case, it was her tendency to worry and to bring her troubles to bedtime. Precipitating factors are stressful life events or illnesses that bring on sleep disturbance. For Jamie, Nanna's hip fracture, her worries for Nanna's health, and the disturbance in her sleep patterns set the stage for worsening sleep.

The third component, perpetuating factors, are efforts to compensate for lost sleep that make the sleep problem worse. Jamie learned that many things she did to cope were perpetuating her insomnia, including caffeine and sleep medication, long afternoon naps, heavy phone use in the late evening, and repeated checking of her clock. Although the allergy medicine helped her sleep at first, it came with "hangover effects" that made her feel groggy the next day; in addition, one can develop tolerance to the sleep-inducing effects of such medicines over time. Collectively, these perpetuating factors led to conditioned arousal, by which the bed and the bedroom became associated with wakefulness rather than sleep.

Her therapist helped her learn many of the techniques of CBT-I, including sleep hygiene, stimulus control, sleep efficiency training, stress management, and especially, that she should trust her body to rediscover its natural sleep skills. Research studies show that CBT-I is as effective as sleep medication in the short term and more effective in the long term, with significantly fewer side effects. For more on CBT-I, see Question 23.

# Glossary

**Adenosine:** An organic compound and byproduct of daytime cellular energy consumption, which is removed from the brain during sleep. As adenosine accumulates across hours of wakefulness, brain activity begins to slow down and feelings of sleepiness develop.

**Advanced Sleep-Wake Phase:** A biological predisposition toward awakening earlier and going to bed earlier than the average individual, sometimes referred to as being a "morning lark" or "early riser." Individuals with advanced circadian rhythms tend to achieve peak mental and physical performance in the morning hours (see Delayed Sleep Phase).

**Caffeine:** One of the most commonly used drugs worldwide that suppresses feelings of sleepiness by blocking brain receptors for adenosine.

**Circadian Rhythm:** A self-sustaining and internally regulated body clock that influences the timing of activity and sleep. The circadian clock is located in a cluster of cells located deep within the brain (i.e., the suprachiasmatic nucleus), which detect light entering the eyes to help synchronize the clock by triggering the release of hormones or suppressing melatonin release.

**Cognitive Behavioral Therapy for Insomnia (CBT-I):** A treatment for insomnia disorder that combines elements of education, sleep hygiene, stimulus control, sleep restriction, stress management, cognitive therapy, and meditation or mindfulness techniques.

**Conditioned Arousal:** A common problem in insomnia disorder where an individual comes to associate the bed or bedroom with wakefulness and frustration, rather than sleep. As a result, getting into bed subtly activates a stress response that overpowers the drive to sleep and increases wakefulness.

**Continuous Positive Airway Pressure (CPAP):** A machine that delivers a steady stream of pressurized room air to a mask placed over the nose or mouth. CPAP is the most effective treatment for obstructive sleep apnea and acts as a pneumatic splint to hold the airway open during sleep to promote normal breathing and sleep.

**Delayed Sleep Phase:** A biological predisposition toward awakening later and going to bed later than the average individual, sometimes referred to as being a "night owl" or "evening type." Individuals with delayed circadian rhythms tend to achieve peak mental and physical performance in the late afternoon or evening (see Advanced Sleep-Wake Phase).

**Gamma-Aminobutyric Acid (GABA):** A neurotransmitter that inhibits the brain's arousal centers, thereby promoting sleep.

**Homeostatic Drive:** A bodily mechanism, also known as the sleep drive, that increases the pressure to sleep the longer an individual remains awake. This occurs as a result of the accumulation of sleep-inducing substances in the brain (e.g., adenosine).

**Insomnia:** A difficulty in falling asleep, having frequent nighttime awakenings, or awakening earlier than intended. Insomnia symptoms are the most common sleep complaint in medical settings.

**Jet Lag:** A temporary difficulty in initiating or maintaining sleep, or daytime effects such as sleepiness, resulting from the circadian rhythm becoming out of sync with local clock time following air travel across time zones.

**Melatonin:** A hormone produced in the pineal gland that aids in regulating circadian sleep timing by promoting sleep.

**Narcolepsy:** A hypersomnolence disorder associated with severe daytime sleepiness, sleep paralysis, and nighttime hallucinations occurring immediately before or after sleep. Type 1 narcolepsy is associated with cataplexy and abnormally low levels or absence of orexin, whereas type 2 narcolepsy typically does not involve cataplexy and is associated with near normal orexin levels.

**Nightmare:** A highly distressing, vivid dream involving perceptions of threat and usually resulting in awakening rapidly with strong dream recall.

**Non-Rapid Eye Movement (NREM) Sleep:** A period of sleep comprised of several sleep stages that gradually transition from wakefulness to sleep onset (stage N1) and from light sleep (stage N2) to deep, slow-wave sleep (stage N3). NREM sleep takes up approximately 75 percent of the total sleep time. In contrast to REM sleep, eye movements and dreams are infrequent in NREM sleep.

**Obstructive Sleep Apnea (OSA):** A sleep-related breathing disorder resulting from a collapse or narrowing of the airway during sleep, particularly between the soft palate and the hard wall at the upper or rear part of the throat, which causes decreased airflow or complete cessation of respiration despite continued efforts to breathe. OSA is one of the most common sleep disorders and interferes with sleep quality, resulting in daytime sleepiness and other medical risks.

**Paralysis:** A loss of muscle control or weakness causing a partial or complete inability to move muscles, such as during REM sleep or waking sleep paralysis.

**Parasomnias:** Abnormal experiences (such as hallucinations or strong emotions) or undesirable behaviors (such as sleepwalking or sleep eating) that occur while asleep or during the transition between sleep and wakefulness. Parasomnias are subdivided as NREM-related, REM-related, and other parasomnias.

**Periodic Limb Movements (PLMs):** Involuntarily movements of the extremities (usually lower limbs) during sleep lasting 0.5–10 seconds in length, which can occur sporadically or in a predictable, repetitive pattern. A diagnosis of periodic limb movement disorder (PLMD) may be considered when movements occur more than 15 times an hour in adults or more than 5 times an hour in children, with associated impairments in sleep quality or daytime functioning.

**Polysomnogram (PSG):** A diagnostic tool and test considered the "gold standard" for the measurement of sleep using sensors attached to the body, which measure physiological changes that naturally occur during sleep (e.g., changes in muscle tension, brain waves, eye movements, breathing and oxygen levels, and heart rate).

**Rapid Eye Movement (REM) Sleep / Stage R:** A stage of sleep taking approximately 25 percent of the total sleep time associated with vivid dreaming and active brain activity, loss of normal muscle tension, and rapid eye movements. One can usually awaken easily from REM sleep and REM increases in frequency and duration toward the end of the sleep period.

**REM Sleep Behavior Disorder (RBD):** A parasomnia marked by a lack of muscle paralysis during REM sleep resulting in the sleeper enacting parts of their dreams, with anything from minor movements to flailing, kicking, speaking or yelling, and aggressive gestures.

**Restless Legs Syndrome (RLS; also known as Willis-Ekbom disease):** A sleep-related movement disorder where unpleasant physical sensations are temporarily relieved by moving the limbs, but the movement delays sleep onset. The sensations occur when at rest in the evening and may be described as "creepy-crawly," "tingling," "itchy," or "electric" sensations deep under the skin.

**Sleep Apnea:** A temporary cessation of normal sleep breathing lasting at least 10 seconds in duration and sometimes associated with awakening or decrease in blood oxygen levels (see Obstructive Sleep Apnea).

**Sleep Hygiene:** A set of lifestyle, environmental, and behavioral recommendations that prevent sleep problems from arising and help promote good quality sleep.

**Sleep-Related Breathing Disorders (SRBD):** A class of sleep disorders associated with difficulties in breathing or abnormal respiration during sleep, which may result in sleep disruption, insufficient oxygen supply, or excessive daytime sleepiness. Sleep apnea is the most common SRBD.

**Sleep-Related Movement Disorders:** A class of sleep disorders associated with repetitive movements that disrupt sleep or prevent sleep onset, such as teeth grinding (nocturnal bruxism) or leg movements as seen in RLS and PLMD.

**Sleep Study:** A diagnostic test for determining the presence of disordered sleep. A sleep study can be either an observed, in-laboratory PSG or conducted remotely using home sleep testing with limited PSG capabilities. A daytime sleep study used to measure sleepiness and diagnose narcolepsy is called the multiple sleep latency test (MSLT) (see Polysomnogram).

**Sleepwalking:** The most common NREM parasomnia, in which sleepwalkers crawl around the bed or walk around their environment with no disturbance in sleep quality.

**Slow-Wave Sleep (SWS) / Stage N3:** A stage of sleep, sometimes referred to as deep sleep, marked by increasingly synchronized and slowed brain activity. People in SWS are difficult to awaken and this stage is most prominent early in the night.

**Stimulus Control:** A set of guidelines within CBT-I that aim to eliminate conditioned arousal by associating the bed with sleep. These recommendations include using the bed for sleep and sex exclusively, going to bed only when feeling sleepy, only sleeping in the bed, and getting out of bed if not sleeping (see Conditioned Arousal).

**Zeitgebers:** A set of external cues that help synchronize the circadian clock, particularly blue spectrum light exposure, timing of exercise and meals, and environmental temperature. From the German word for "time giver."

# Directory of Resources

## BOOKS

Alexandre, R. (2020). *The Sleep Workbook: Easy Strategies to Break the Anxiety-Insomnia Cycle.* Rockridge Press.

Carney, C. E., & Manber, R. (2009). *Quiet Your Mind & Get to Sleep.* New Harbinger Publications.

Carney, C. E., & Manber, R. (2013). *Goodnight Mind: Turn Off Your Noisy Thoughts and Get a Good Night's Sleep.* New Harbinger Publications.

Kryger, M. H., Roth, T., & Dement, W. C. (2016). *Principles and Practice of Sleep Medicine.* 6th Edition. Elsevier.

Walker, M. (2017). *Why We Sleep: Unlocking the Power of Sleep and Dreams.* Scribner Books.

## ORGANIZATIONS

**American Academy of Sleep Medicine**
2510 North Frontage Road
Darien, IL 60561
(630) 737-9700
Fax: (630) 737-9790
https://www.aasm.org/
The only professional organization dedicated exclusively to the medical subspecialty of sleep medicine.

**American Sleep Apnea Association**
1250 Connecticut Ave NW Ste 700
Washington, DC 20036
888-293-3650
http://www.sleepapnea.org
Organization providing educational materials, services, research, and advocacy to improve the lives of people with sleep apnea.

**American Sleep Association**
100 Cambridge Street, Suite 1400
Boston, MA 02114
https://www.sleepassociation.org/
Advocacy and educational organization led by physicians and scientists to increase awareness of the importance of sleep and sleep disorders.

**Circadian Sleep Disorders Network**
4619 Woodfield Rd.
Bethesda, MD 20814
http://www.circadiansleepdisorders.org
Organization providing education and advocacy for accommodations in education and employment for people with circadian rhythm sleep disorders.

**Narcolepsy Network**
PO Box 2178
Lynnwood, WA 98036
(888) 292-6522
https://narcolepsynetwork.org/
Patient support organization providing education, support, and advocacy for narcolepsy patients, family, friends, medical providers, and the general public.

**National Sleep Foundation**
1010 N. Glebe Road, Suite 310
Arlington, VA 22201
(703) 243-1697
https://www.sleepfoundation.org/
Organization whose mission is to improve health and well-being through sleep education and advocacy. The National Sleep Foundation conducts the Sleep in America poll and spearheads initiatives to increase public and medical professional awareness on sleep.

**Restless Legs Syndrome Foundation**
3006 Bee Caves Road, Suite D206

Austin, Texas 78746
(512) 366-9109
https://www.rls.org/
Organization dedicated to improving the lives of people with restless legs syndrome and providing support, education, and research.

**Society of Behavioral Sleep Medicine**
1522 Player Drive
Lexington, KY 40511
(859) 312-8880
Fax: (859) 303-6055
https://www.behavioralsleep.org/
An interdisciplinary organization committed to advancing the scientific approach to studying the behavioral, psychological, and physiological dimensions of sleep; includes a useful provider search directory.

**Wake Up Narcolepsy: Advocacy Organization Website**
http://www.wakeupnarcolepsy.org
Website with information on narcolepsy and its treatment for an organization involved in fundraising, grant distribution, and engagement with the patient community.

## WEBSITES

**American Academy of Sleep Medicine. (2023).**
http://sleepeducation.org/
An educational website on sleep and sleep disorders. Also provides a free sleep diary resource to graphically track sleep over a two-week period, which is particularly helpful when assessing Circadian Rhythm Sleep-wake Disorders. https://sleepeducation.org/docs/default-document-library/sleep-diary.pdf

**National Highway Traffic Safety Administration. (2020). U.S. Department of Transportation.**
https://www.nhtsa.gov/risky-driving/drowsy-driving
Website with information relating to the dangers of drowsy driving.

**National Sleep Foundation. (2020). Sleep Diary.**
https://www.sleepfoundation.org/sites/default/files/inline-files/SleepDiaryv6.pdf
A free one-week sleep log, tracking sleep timing variables, mood, medication and substance use, daytime sleepiness, and sleep hygiene factors.

**U.S. Department of Veterans Affairs (VA). (2019). CBT-i Coach (Version 2.4) [Mobile application software].**
https://apps.apple.com/us/app/cbt-i-coach/id655918660
A free, easy-to-use mobile application for people who have experienced symptoms of insomnia and would like to improve their sleep habits; includes a sleep diary, recommendations to improve sleep, and relaxation tools.

**WGBH Educational Foundation and the Harvard Medical School Division of Sleep Medicine. (2008, January 2). Healthy Sleep: Understanding the Third of Our Lives We So Often Take for Granted.**
http://healthysleep.med.harvard.edu/
A free resource with videos and interactive activities that aims to help the general public understand the science of sleep and provides practical guidance on achieving healthy sleep.

# Index

## About the Authors

**John T. Peachey**, PsyD, is a medical psychologist and coauthor of *What You Need to Know about Sleep Disorders*. He was selected as a William C. Dement Fellow for sleep research, completed a fellowship in behavioral sleep medicine at Stanford University's School of Medicine, and has worked internationally in military behavioral medicine.

**Diane C. Zelman**, PhD, is a professor in the PhD program in clinical psychology at Alliant International University's California School of Professional Psychology in the San Francisco Bay Area, California. She is also an assistant clinical professor in the Department of Family and Community Medicine at the University of California, San Francisco. She coauthored *What You Need to Know about Sleep Disorders* and has published extensively on topics in health psychology, particularly in studies of sleep, chronic pain, and addiction.